HEART

9-5-08
you did great,
congratulations!
Good luck.
(signature)

9/13/08

To Mr. Householder,
with best wishes
for future health,

John

ADVANCE PRAISE

"Your Heart: An Owner's Guide is an excellent contribution to the patient-care literature that not only informs but enlightens patients and family members. I particularly enjoy the case presentations and the patient-friendly language."

—Robert S. D. Higgins, MD, MSHA, The Mary and John Bent Professor and Chair, Department of Cardiovascular and Thoracic Surgery, Rush University Medical Center, Chicago, IL

"Both Dr. Elefteriades and Dr. Cohen are consummate clinicians. Their book addresses every question a patient could ask of a cardiovascular specialist."

—Michael D. Ezekowitz, MD, PhD, Professor and Vice President, Lankenau Institute for Medical Research; Cardiologist, CASEP Medical Group, Wynnewood, PA

"Your Heart: An Owner's Guide is an outstanding resource for heart patients and their families. It contains answers to most all of the questions patients ask their cardiologists and cardiac surgeons in the office, as well as to the questions patients may not ask but later wish they had. It covers the most basic principles of heart anatomy and disease, as well as more sophisticated concepts of how cardiac surgery is performed. Readers will learn the reasons behind the tests and the treatments doctors recommend, and they will better understand what patients can and should do to improve their own heart health."

—Eric M. Isselbacher, MD, Associate Director, Massachusetts General Hospital Heart Center

YOUR
HEART
An Owner's Guide

JOHN A. ELEFTERIADES, MD
LAWRENCE S. COHEN, MD
Foreword by ROBERT JARVIK, MD

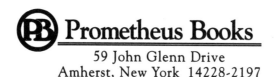 Prometheus Books
59 John Glenn Drive
Amherst, New York 14228-2197

Published 2007 by Prometheus Books

Inquiries should be addressed to
Prometheus Books
59 John Glenn Drive
Amherst, New York 14228–2197
VOICE: 716–691–0133, ext. 207
FAX: 716–564–2711
WWW.PROMETHEUSBOOKS.COM

11 10 09 08 07 06   5 4 3 2 1

Library of Congress Cataloging-in-Publication Data

Elefteriades, John A.
    Your heart : an owner's guide / by John A. Elefteriades and Lawrence S. Cohen.
       p. cm.
    Includes bibliographical references and index.
    ISBN 978–1–59102–451–4 (alk. paper)
    1. Heart—Diseases—Miscellanea. 2. Heart—Miscellanea. I. Cohen, Lawrence S.
II. Title.

RC682.E384 2007
616.1'2—dc22

2006035312

Printed in the United States on acid-free paper

For our patients,
from whom we have learned and
from whom we have received
more than we have given.

TABLE OF CONTENTS

ACKNOWLEDGMENTS

The authors wish to acknowledge certain individuals for their contributions to the development of this book.

We wish to thank Ms. Susan Schulman for her encouragement and advice in the early stages of this work.

We express sincere gratitude to Ms. Rosalie Siegel, of the Rosalie Siegel Agency, for her wisdom and expertise, which brought this manuscript to fruition. We also thank Ms. Linda Regan, of Prometheus Books, for her superb editorial input.

The authors express their most sincere appreciation to the extremely talented Ms. Alexandra Baker of DNA Illustrations (New Orleans, LA) for her superb work in illustrating this book. We feel that the illustrations constitute an important part of the value of this book to the reader.

Sincere thanks go to Mary Ann Tranquilli, RN, who applied her wealth of experience with patients and their families in suggesting extremely helpful improvements in the content of this book.

Thanks go as well to Ms. Rhaea Miller and Ms. Marianne McCarthy for their administrative assistance and to Ms. Christina Elefteriades for her copyediting.

The authors would like to thank John Breslin, RN, and George Tolis, MD, for applying their photographic talents in the operating room.

Special thanks go to Mr. and Mrs. Sheridan, an open heart surgery patient and his wife with considerable language skills, who reviewed the manuscript in detail and made very helpful suggestions.

We also wish to thank our patients, thousands upon thousands of them, whom it has been our privilege to attend. It is our patients

10   ACKNOWLEDGMENTS

who have asked the very pertinent questions addressed in this book. Nearly all of these questions have arisen in real-life clinical situations with our patients.

FOREWORD

By Dr. Robert Jarvik

Someone close to you has heart disease. Someone you know well. Someone you love. And someone who was close has died from heart disease.

What about you? You know your heart is in danger.

Do you know enough about the most common health risk we all face?

Your Heart: An Owner's Guide will help you, because the more you understand about your heart and modern cardiac medicine, the better decisions you will make about your health. Do you know your risk factors for heart disease? What tests should you have? Do you understand what your doctor recommends for you?

Do you know what you can do to reduce your risk? Do you have high blood pressure? Are you obese? Is your blood cholesterol excessive? Are you exercising enough? Have you stopped smoking yet?!

Our knowledge about preventing heart disease continues to increase, but as more and more results of large clinical studies are reported to the public, knowing what to do doesn't necessarily become more clear. Some of the things the public has believed for years are proving to be wrong, like the idea that reducing the percentage of fat in your diet helps prevent heart disease, stroke, and some forms of cancer.

This book gives you detailed information about heart disease, its prevention and its treatment, explained clearly by two outstanding specialists, a cardiologist and a heart surgeon from Yale. They answer in a clear style most of the questions patients commonly ask, which gives you the facts in a way you can understand.

And the more you understand, the stronger you will be if you have heart disease and need to deal with serious illness.

These days people don't read most books to the end, except perhaps novels and thrillers. They read parts of books. They skim them looking for special information. You could do that with *Your Heart*, because you might be particularly interested in a certain topic, like valve surgery if you need a heart valve operation. But the more of *Your Heart* you read, the more you will understand about your heart and why heart specialists do what we do. You will learn something of interest, and something important in every chapter.

Your Heart is clear. It is easy to understand, and its particular advantage is that it gives you an expert medical overview by doctors who understand patients as people, and heart disease as medical science.

Learn as much as you can from this book. You need to know.

Robert Jarvik, MD
President and CEO
Jarvik Heart, Inc.
New York, New York

PREFACE

We wish to say, "Welcome to our office." We hope that you treat this encounter with our book like a visit to the doctor. Whether you or your loved one suffers from congenital heart disease, coronary heart disease, valvular heart disease, heart failure, and/or arrhythmias, you will find information on these problems right here. Perhaps the personal story of one of the patients we present in the "clinical vignettes" in this book will strike very close to home. You may even feel like it is you or your loved one being described. We want this book to be like an office visit with a heart specialist.

We hope and suspect that the questions we pose and answer in this book reflect actual questions that you may have or that arise in your mind as you learn more about heart disease.

In this era of managed health care, the amount of time that even a dedicated heart specialist can devote to a single patient encounter is often limited. This book offers you essentially an unlimited office visit. You can read and learn all you want to know about your cardiac problem. Plus, the answers and information are illustrated and written down for you, so you can refer back to them. We are all aware that so much of the information offered in traditional patient visits is hard to assimilate or to remember. We are glad the information in this book is complete and well documented so that you can review it again and again, extracting more specific details and understanding more fully with each review.

Heart disease is estimated to affect nearly sixty million Americans—one in every six of us. Nearly three-quarters of a million people die in our country each year from heart disease. Virtually every family in the country has or has had a family member affected by one of the many afflictions that can attack the heart. These millions of patients and their family members want and need comprehensive information in an understandable format.

Throughout this book, we specifically address questions that we hear every day from our patients with heart disease. We include only that medical background information that is necessary for a complete answer to the question at hand. There is no need to provide page after page of anatomy and pathology jargon to give specific answers to your concerns.

As your authors, we—a cardiothoracic surgeon and a cardiologist—have immense hands-on experience in taking care of patients. We know what concerns are foremost in patients' minds. These concerns specifically and exclusively inform the questions posed and answered in this book.

Although you may so choose, you do not need to read this book in sequence from cover to cover. You should feel free to use the table of contents, the index, and the lists of illustrations and case vignettes to help you locate the sections of special importance to you. You may recognize your own situation or even your own questions in one or more of the vignettes. We suggest that you use the specific question headings to locate information that is essential to you in understanding or deciding about your cardiac care or that of your family member. You may well find that just by leafing through this book, you are drawn to information of particular interest by headings, questions, and figures that reflect your own circumstances. In our efforts to provide easy access to specific information, we may have included some overlap between different questions and answers. We have done this to provide you with as comprehensive an answer as possible without your having to search back and forth throughout the book. We hope that by using the book in this way, it will become your "owner's guide" to your own heart.

We included numerous illustrations and diagrams of anatomy,

medical devices, surgical techniques and tools, as well as photographs of operating room scenes. The figures themselves tell much of the story of cardiac illness and the available treatments. The figures can also focus your attention on corresponding text of relevance to a problem or decision that you or your loved one is facing.

For ease of reading, we have used the male pronoun when referring to heart specialists, though we are thrilled that women are increasingly represented among cardiologists and heart surgeons. Likewise, we have usually chosen the male pronoun for referring to patients; please note, however, that we have devoted an entire chapter specifically to heart disease in women.

We hope you enjoy your journey through the information in this book and that you may be rewarded by greater understanding of cardiac function, cardiac disease, and the available treatments.

John A. Elefteriades, MD
Professor and Chief of Cardiothoracic Surgery
Yale University School of Medicine
New Haven, Connecticut

Lawrence S. Cohen, MD
Ebenezer K. Hunt Professor of Cardiology
Yale University School of Medicine
New Haven, Connecticut

INTRODUCTION TO THE HEART

Your heart is one remarkable muscle. Just think about the simple fact that this muscle contracts every minute of every day for your entire life. Can you imagine any other muscle in your body contracting continuously without rest? Can you do push-ups ad infinitum? How about sit-ups? Not likely. Can you run continuously without stopping? Definitely not. Not even the world's best and most highly trained athletes can persuade any of their skeletal muscles (those that move the limbs) to work incessantly without rest. No other muscle is as tireless or has the same capability as your heart. The heart muscle has unique innate cellular and metabolic characteristics that permit it to function continuously and without rest.

You might say, how about my diaphragm? Don't I breathe all day, every day? The diaphragm does share some of the heart's tirelessness. However, only small and varying bundles of the diaphragm muscle fibers contract at any one time. The brain varies the contracting bundles continuously from breath to breath, allowing those not in use to rest. Not even the very powerful diaphragm muscle is as tireless as the heart. In the heart, each and every muscle cell contracts with each and every heartbeat, as remarkable as this may seem. (Your brain certainly works full time, but the brain is a collection of nerve cells, not a contracting muscle.)

For all this muscle activity, the heart needs blood flow, and lots of it. A network of arteries on the surface of the heart—the coronary arteries—carries blood flow to the heart muscle itself. The oxygen and nutrients delivered to the heart muscle give your heart the energy to pump the blood within its chambers to the rest of the body. The word coronary derives from "corona," or "crown." To early anatomists, the coronary artery network resembled a thin crown draped over the heart.

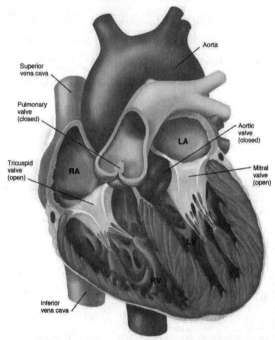

Figure 1. An overview of the heart's anatomy.

Like any other mechanical pump, the heart needs valves to keep blood flowing forward. The pumping chambers of the heart require an inflow valve and an outflow valve. Without an inflow valve, blood already in the heart could leak backward, against the bloodstream. Without an outflow valve, blood already propelled forward would come right back to the heart. The proverbial Sisyphus of Greek mythology was cursed to push a heavy stone up a hill only to keep repeating this action each time it rolled down. The same would be true for your poor heart without an outflow valve—it would push a heartful of blood forward, only to have it come right back again, to be propelled yet once more.

The powerful pumping chamber of the heart is called the ventricle. The ventricle that pumps to the rest of your body is the left ventricle. It pumps blood to your head, your arms, your liver, your intestines, your legs, and virtually all organs of your body. The walls of the left ventricle are about one to two centimeters thick (about a half to one inch). This chamber pumps about five quarts of blood every minute, which requires an energy equivalent to about that used by an 80-watt lightbulb. When an athlete is at peak exertion, his heart can pump ten or even twelve quarts of blood per minute.

You can follow the events of the cardiac cycle in the figure below.

Leading into the left ventricle is the left atrium. The left atrium collects the blood coming back from the lungs and channels it into the powerful left ventricle. The left atrium, unlike the ventricle, is thin-walled. It imparts only a small "boost" to the blood that it propels into the left ventricle. We liken the atrial chamber to the "turbocharger" of a high-performance car engine. It loads the main engine under pressure, thus improving its power output. The atrium boosts the output of your left ventricle by about one-fifth. The phase of the cardiac cycle during which the left ventricle is inactive, and being loaded, is called *diastole*. It is the left ventricle that provides the powerful burst of squeezing action that propels the blood around the body. This phase of the cardiac cycle—when the left ventricle is contracting and ejecting blood—is called systole. During the interval between one systole and the next, the heart rests, recovers, and fills passively with blood, preparing for the next active heartbeat.

Up to this point, we have discussed only the left atrium and the left ventricle—the so-called left side of the heart. As you will recall, your heart also has a right side. The responsibility of the "right heart" is to pump blood to the lungs. That is the one and only responsibility for the right heart. As you might imagine, this does

Diastole

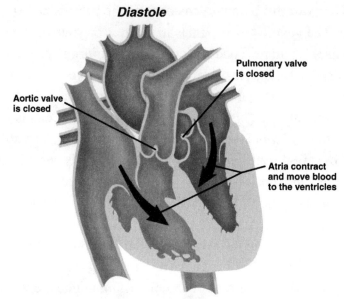

Figures 2a and 2b. The events of the cardiac cycle. Part a (above) shows the passive phase of the left ventricle, in which it is loading with blood. This is called diastole. Part b (below) shows the active contracting phase of the left ventricle, called systole.

Systole

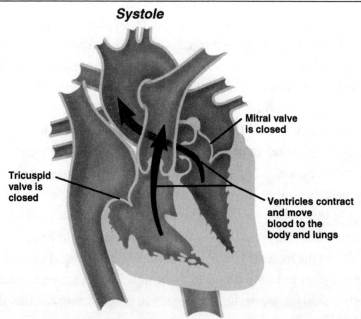

not require as much power as is necessary for the left heart. Accordingly, the right ventricle is thin, about half a centimeter (a quarter inch) and expends about 20 watts of energy. The right ventricle has its own auxiliary atrium, called the right atrium. The right atrium boosts the blood entering the right ventricle. The right atrium collects all the blood coming back from the body and channels it into the right ventricle, for delivery to the lungs.

So, let's track a single drop of blood through your circulation. Let's watch it on its way to a target organ, say, your brain. (We could pick any organ or muscle in your body.) Under pressure from the heart, the drop of blood enters your brain and supplies the oxygen and nutrients to allow your brain to function—that is, to maintain your consciousness and allow you to read this book, for example. After passing through your brain, the blood passes along the veins of your body back to the right atrium. The right atrium gives the drop of blood a little mechanical boost and channels it into the right ventricle. The right ventricle propels the droplet into your lungs, where it picks up oxygen from the air you breathe.

From your lungs, the drop of blood enters the left atrium, which gives it a boost into the left ventricle. The muscle-bound left ventricle—the main powerhouse of the heart—propels this drop of blood out again to your body, thus completing the repetitive circuit.

This book is intended to help you understand the function of your heart, both in health and in disease. The heart can make its trouble known to the patient in a variety of ways. From the case histories, the questions and answers, and the illustrations in this book, it is our desire that you gain considerable understanding of heart disease—including its causes, diagnosis, treatment, and outlook.

In general, patients with heart disease may experience symptoms of inadequate blood flow to the heart muscle, symptoms of congestive heart failure, and symptoms of arrhythmia (altered rhythm) of the heart. Inadequate blood flow is usually felt as chest pain. Congestive heart failure is usually experienced as shortness of breath. Altered rhythms of the heart are felt as severe light-headedness or loss of consciousness. The most serious symptom of heart disease is cardiac arrest, which in earlier times was almost always fatal, but in this era of a highly educated public is more often successfully treated.

Patients are seeking more and more information about their heart disease and the options for treating it. They want to know why they contracted their disease. They want to know what they can do to prevent its progression. They want to know which medications they should be taking. And, in severe cases, they want to know what procedures can be performed either in the catheterization laboratory or in the operating room. In anticipating such procedures, they wish to know what the dangers may be as well as what potential benefits may reasonably be expected.

In this book, we are attempting to take you virtually *inside* the consultation room. We hope you feel that you are essentially sitting in front of the expert's desk and asking all the questions that you have.

We hope and expect that the information available in this book will supplement the discussions you have with your own doctors. No physician could possibly take the time necessary to provide all the information and answers contained here.

Finally, this book is not intended only for patients. We hope it will be of use as well to concerned family members. Increasingly, we find our consultation rooms full of adult children of patients with heart disease who are eager to know the outlook for their parents and how to aid them in their decision making. These children are often very well informed and eager for in-depth additional knowledge. We hope that virtually all pieces of information that a patient or family could reasonably wish to receive will be contained herein. New, emerging, and cutting-edge technologies are covered comprehensively in the sections corresponding to their applications. The organization into chapters, the patient question headings, and the index should help patients and families to find the specific information they want without undue time and effort.

The organization around specific questions, grouped into chapters, will permit returning to the book in split sessions whenever time is available. Again, there need be no concern to read cover to cover consecutively.

We sincerely hope that the information in this book will help you to understand your or your family member's heart disease, to do all that you can to prevent its progression, and to select diagnostic studies and treatments wisely. It is assumed, of course, that this information will be used only to supplement information and advice you personally receive from your treating physicians.

Disclaimer. This book is not intended to permit you to diagnose or to treat yourself, nor is it intended to supplant in any way the interaction between you and your physician. The purposes of this book are to provide you some background knowledge with which to understand your heart condition better and to augment the information that your physician can supply in the time you spend together. Although most of the information presented in this book is relatively mainstream, representing standard medical understandings and policies, differences of opinion may exist on specific issues. Your care is and should be entrusted to your physician.

CORONARY ARTERY DISEASE

Case 1: Trouble in the Cherry Picker.

Robert hadn't been sick a day in his life. Sure, he had put on some pounds over the years, mainly around his middle, but at fifty-five, he was still fit enough to climb utility poles every day as a repairman for the phone company. One night, he didn't feel quite right. He was tired and took several heartburn tablets from his medicine cabinet. He was able to get to sleep, and felt fine when he got up in the morning. Later, when he had a 20,000-volt line disconnected and was suspended thirty feet in the air in his cherry picker, he knew he was in trouble. He felt a pain right in the middle of his chest. He could have sworn that an elephant had sat right there on top of his sternum. He felt light-headed. He sat back in the cherry picker and thought he would have to vomit right over the side.

Fortunately, on this day, he was out with a partner. Back in the truck cab, Marty sensed right away that something was wrong with Robert. He brought the cherry picker down, and didn't like what he saw. Robert was pale. He was sweating profusely, although it was a cool autumn day. His breathing was obviously heavy, labored. Marty had to rouse his partner to get him to tocus his eyes. Marty phoned the ambulance immediately, which arrived within minutes. It looked like a heart attack, the medics told Marty. It was good he had called right away. Marty saw the medics put an oxygen mask on Robert's face. They started an IV and ran some "nitro." As the ambulance pulled away, Marty thought Robert looked better.

Later that night, Marty visited Robert in the coronary care unit—the CCU, as it is called. Sally and the kids were there. Robert was sitting up in bed, picking at his dinner. Sally expressed her thanks for Marty's concern and prompt action out in the field. She explained that the doctors had told her that Robert had had a severe angina attack. Without prompt attention, it would have progressed to a heart attack. The oxygen, the nitroglycerine, and the blood thinner heparin, as well as an aspirin tablet, had succeeded in turning things around. The heart attack had been aborted. The EKG (electrocardiogram) had returned to normal.

Robert would need a catheterization, though. The doctors were sure he had coronary artery disease—blockages in the coronary arteries, which supply blood to the heart muscle itself.

What is angina?

Most people are familiar with angina, the overt manifestation of inadequate flow of blood to the heart. Angina was first described by the British physician William Heberden more than two hundred years ago. Figure 1.1, adapted from the Netter series, a well-known collection of anatomical illustrations used to train doctors, shows the areas of pain in a typical patient with angina.

The heart is a muscle. As such, it requires blood flow and oxygen delivery in order to function. In contrast to other muscles

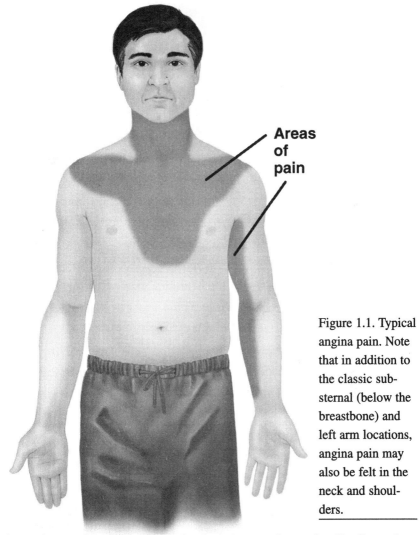

**Areas
of
pain**

Figure 1.1. Typical angina pain. Note that in addition to the classic sub-sternal (below the breastbone) and left arm locations, angina pain may also be felt in the neck and shoulders.

throughout the body, which function only episodically when needed, the heart pumps "twenty-four/seven" throughout our lives. Even a period of seconds without heart function leads to unconsciousness and threat of organ damage. The diaphragm, the large muscle used for breathing, which separates the chest from the abdomen, is the other muscle in the body that operates full time, all the time. In the case of the heart, its blood flow and oxygen requirements are huge. The heart requires about one cup of blood per minute to nourish itself at rest. Under stress, it can utilize over one quart of blood per minute just to meet its own nutrient needs. This corresponds to about one-fifth of the total baseline flow of blood in the body. Even a short interruption of blood flow to the heart muscle itself will lead to oxygen deprivation of the heart cells. If this does not last more than a few minutes, no permanent damage to these cells is incurred. The transiently insufficient blood flow is felt as typical angina pain. The classic characteristics of this pain are that it is felt *substernally*, under the breastbone, and that it is perceived as a *pressurelike* pain. The classic scenario is that of a patient clutching his chest in severe discomfort. The pain is often described in terms such as the following: "I feel like an elephant is sitting on my chest." "I feel like I have a vise on my chest." The patient often uses a clenched fist over his chest to illustrate what he is feeling.

Angina is really the muscle burn that one can feel from any muscle stressed to the point of exceeding its blood flow capacity. For example, you can do sit-ups to the point of exhaustion. The intense pain you will feel in your midsection is really "angina," so to speak, of your abdominal muscles.

We grade your angina according to the level of exertion required to bring it on. This is called the Canadian Cardiovascular Society classification system. If the patient has no angina whatsoever, despite exertion, he is Class I. If angina comes on only with vigorous exertion (at the gym, for example), he is Class II. If the angina comes on with only mild exertion (as in walking on level ground), he is Class III. If the angina comes on with no exertion, during the resting state, the angina is the highest category, or Class IV. Class IV patients may feel angina while resting, watching TV, reading, or even sleeping.

Severe anginal attacks, especially those likely to eventuate in a heart attack, may be accompanied by profuse sweating. Friends or relatives may comment on an ashen color or an appearance of obvious physical distress.

Doctors used to think that all or most patients with inadequate blood flow to the heart would feel angina pain. We now know that many patients, perhaps up to 40 percent, do not feel angina pain. This may be dangerous for a number of reasons. First, these patients may escape diagnosis of their heart disease entirely. Second, even patients with known heart disease may not be aware when they are exceeding their heart's capacity. After all, symptoms of disease, in general, reflect the body's intrinsic "early warning system." Patients who do not feel angina have a defective warning system. Such a defective pain mechanism is seen especially in diabetic patients, in whom the sensory nerves are damaged by the excess ambient sugar levels in the body.

What is the cause of angina?

As explained above, angina occurs when the heart muscle's demand for oxygen is greater than the supply. Pain fibers in the muscle are stimulated, and angina occurs. The root cause of angina is blockages in the coronary arteries, which are responsible for supplying oxygen-rich blood to the heart muscle itself.

Typically, anginal pain comes on with exertion. The reason for this is that in the resting state, even with blockages in the arteries that deliver blood flow to the heart, the delivery of blood and oxygen is adequate to meet the heart's needs. As exertion proceeds, the heart needs more and more oxygen, and the blocked arteries cannot deliver the required levels. Patients often first notice heart pain, or angina, during bursts of severe exertion, such as running for a bus or hurrying between terminals at the airport.

Other states that can trigger angina, by increasing oxygen

demands in the heart above the available delivery, include stress and anxiety. A patient may feel anginal discomfort during an intense marital dispute or during a stressful meeting at work.

Common activities may increase the demand for oxygen and cause angina. Jogging, walking briskly up the stairs, or getting overheated while watching an exciting sporting event may be the precipitant. Any activity that causes the heart to beat more rapidly or causes the blood pressure to rise may trigger angina. Oxygen demand may also exceed supply after a big meal, when blood and oxygen are diverted from the heart to the intestinal tract. An easy way to remember the major causes of angina is to think of the three E's: exercise, emotion, and eating.

These are classic descriptions of typical angina. As all experienced physicians know, the manifestations of angina can vary greatly. Angina is not always felt in the typical substernal, or mid-chest, location. It may be felt in the left arm or shoulder. It may be felt in the jaw. Rarely, it may be felt in the back or in the teeth or neck. On occasion, it may be felt as a heartburn-type discomfort, easily confused with symptoms of dyspepsia originating in the nearly ubiquitous acid reflux that most adults experience at some times. Especially in women, anginal symptoms may be atypical (see Chapter 14).

Characteristically, anginal pain disappears when the exertion ends, as the demands of the heart for blood and oxygen come down within the limits that can be provided by the diseased arteries. Typically, angina goes away within a minute or two of sitting down and resting.

My doctor says I have "angina at rest." What does that mean?

Usually anginal attacks are brought on by specific activities above the particular patient's threshold for exertion. Often patients know that, on their daily walk, for example, pain will come on precisely two-thirds of the way up a certain hill. Sometimes, instead of phys-ical exertion, the cause for a specific bout of angina may be emo-tion or a heavy meal, both of which can tax the heart. When pain comes on without any exertion or other provocation, we call that *angina at rest*. This is an important sign because angina at rest may predict that a heart attack is imminent.

If you are getting chest pains when you are resting, seated com-fortably, perhaps while reading or watching TV, you may have angina at rest. This is a potentially serious pattern, which you should promptly call to the attention of your doctor.

How many coronary arteries do I have?

The coronary arteries originate directly above the aortic valve. There, two coronary arteries arise from the aorta and course over the heart like a crown or corona. This is why they are called *coro-nary arteries*. See figure 1.2 below.

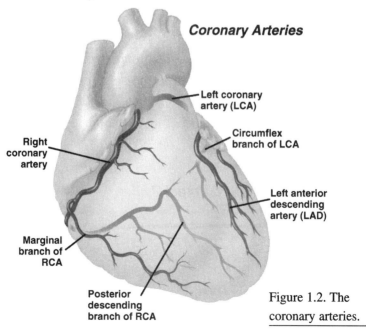

Figure 1.2. The coronary arteries.

The left coronary artery divides into two branches shortly after its beginning, becoming the left anterior descending artery and the left circumflex coronary artery. The left anterior descending coronary artery runs over the front surface of the heart, and the left circumflex coronary artery distributes itself over the lateral surface of the heart. The left anterior descending coronary artery (or LAD) is by far the most important artery of the heart, supplying by itself over 40 percent of the total blood flow to the heart.

The other major coronary artery is the right coronary artery. In general, it supplies blood to the back surface of the heart.

What is coronary artery disease?

Coronary artery disease refers to the buildup of fatty deposits in the wall of one of the arteries that supplies blood to the heart. This buildup narrows the central channel of the artery, decreasing the amount of blood and oxygen that can be carried to the heart muscle. The process of coronary arteriosclerosis, hardening of the arteries of the heart from fatty deposits, takes decades to develop. Coronary arteriosclerosis is defined as the development of narrowings in the coronary arteries due to buildup of fatty plaques. Coronary artery plaques are composed of cholesterol fats, circulating cells from the bloodstream, and tissue cells reacting to the presence of all of these elements.

What causes a heart attack?

The process of arteriosclerosis usually occurs gradually, resulting in a pattern of regular angina. In some cases, a sudden adverse event occurs, triggering a heart attack. This sudden adverse event occurs as follows.

If a plaque ruptures into the lumen, or central channel, of a coronary artery, this material gets exposed to the bloodstream. The nature of this material causes clotting of blood that streams past it. As the blood clot, or thrombus, grows, it starts to block or occlude the coronary artery at the site of the plaque rupture. The expanding clot does not allow blood to flow by it, thereby depriving part of the heart muscle of blood and oxygen.

As this process extends into many minutes or hours, some of the heart muscle, deprived of oxygen, begins to die. Death of heart muscle is the definition of a heart attack. (Angina alone does not do this.) If blood flow is not fairly promptly restored, the dead muscle is forever lost and forms a scar. We usually use the standard of four hours—if blood flow is not restored within this window of time, at least some of the affected muscle will die. This process is depicted in the accompanying figure.

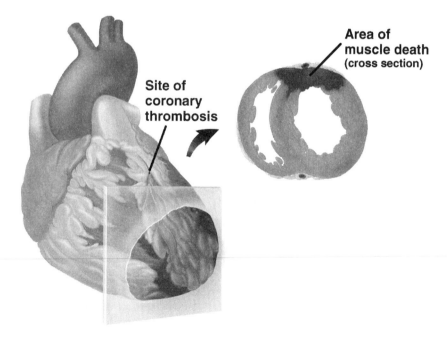

Figure 1.3. A completed heart attack.

What are the symptoms of a heart attack?

The classic symptom of a heart attack is severe chest pain, which may be localized to the breastbone area or, in some patients, may radiate to the arms, shoulders, back, jaw, or upper abdomen. Pain in the left arm is very common. Generally, there is a feeling of significant generalized weakness and a foreboding of doom. Sweating is common. Although the pain is often quite severe, the level of pain may vary. In women, the pain may be minor or absent, with nausea predominating, as we will discuss in chapter 14. The pain may be intermittent, as the culprit clot may also undergo variable degrees of dissolution by the body's own reparative mechanisms.

Can gall bladder problems simulate heart disease?

It is not always simple to localize the site of pain. Although gall bladder symptoms typically occur on the right side of the upper abdomen, under the rib cage, the discomfort can at times occur in the chest. Usually, the relation of gall bladder symptoms to meals, especially fatty ones, helps to lead to the correct diagnosis of an abdominal, rather than a cardiac, problem.

In some cases, the symptoms of the two organs, gall bladder and heart, can even mimic each other. Certain characteristics can help to distinguish the two diseases. The person who develops gall bladder disease often has a distinctive profile. It is said that the typical candidate is "female, fifty, fertile, overweight, and fair-complexioned." Although exceptions obviously occur, the index of suspicion rises the more closely the patient with symptoms approaches the classic description. In any case, a simple ultrasound exam will show conclusively whether or not you have gallstones.

How can I tell if it is an anginal episode or if I am suffering a heart attack?

There are some distinguishing characteristics between an anginal episode and a heart attack (also known as a coronary thrombosis).

First and foremost is the duration of symptoms. An anginal episode usually subsides within a few minutes. Pain that lasts beyond twenty minutes is considered to be a heart attack in evolution.

Another distinguishing characteristic is the relation of the pain to exertion. An anginal episode goes away when the exertion stops. Not so a heart attack. The pain of a heart attack continues even after the exertion has stopped.

Another characteristic has to do with the response to a nitroglycerine tablet. An anginal episode will subside promptly with the first or second nitro. The pain from a heart attack, however, continues despite nitroglycerine. The pain usually does not go away until morphine is administered in the hospital.

The pain of a heart attack usually comes on suddenly, reflecting the sudden occlusion of a coronary artery. Anginal pain, on the other hand, is more gradual in onset, as exertion increases the oxygen demand of the heart muscle above what the coronary arteries can supply.

A patient having a heart attack may sense what we call a feeling of impending doom, an intuitive sense that his or her life is in severe danger. This does not usually characterize an anginal episode.

A heart attack is often accompanied by other symptoms, such as nausea, vomiting, and severe sweating. Friends, family, or coworkers may note an ashen color. These additional symptoms and signs are less common with an uncomplicated anginal attack.

The following table indicates some of these differentiating features.

If in any doubt at all, you should dial 911 and be taken immediately to the hospital's emergency room. The EKG will usually make it immediately clear if you are experiencing a heart attack.

Table 1.1. Features of Angina and Heart Attack.		
	Angina	*Heart Attack*
Duration	one or two minutes	greater than twenty minutes
Relation to exertion	Subsides with cessation	Does not subside despite cessation
Response to TNG (trinitro glycerine)	Responds well	Does not respond
Onset	Gradual	Sudden
Sense of "doom"	Not usually	Often
Associated symptoms and signs	Not usually	Nausea, vomiting, sweating, ashen color

Do I have to be concerned if I get pain in my left arm when I exercise but get none in my chest?

The pain during angina usually begins in the center of the chest and then radiates to the shoulders and down the inside of the left arm. This is the classic presentation. However, there may well be variations of this pattern. At times it may radiate to the jaw and be confused with a toothache. In other cases, it may be felt exclusively in the left arm. Angina generally lasts for a few minutes and subsides when the person stops the activity and rests. Any chest pain that is brought on by exertion and goes away when that activity is stopped must raise the suspicion that angina is present. A doctor's visit is warranted.

What are some of the other causes of chest pain that are not angina?

There are a myriad of other causes of chest pain that are not due to a coronary artery problem. Gall bladder disease has been mentioned. Hiatus hernia, where the upper portion of the stomach has situated itself above the diaphragm is another. Esophagitis or esophageal spasm may cause chest pain. A peptic ulcer may at times be confused with other causes of chest pain. Musculoskeletal pain or cervical spine disease may radiate to the chest. Patients with mitral valve prolapse (an excess mobility of the mitral valve common in young women) often complain of chest pain. An inflammation of the lining surrounding the heart, pericarditis, may cause chest pain (see chapter 12). States of anxiety are at times the cause of perceived chest pain. More serious causes of chest pain may include a blood clot in the lungs, called a *pulmonary embolus*, or a dissecting aneurysm of the ascending aorta. See the accompanying list.

CAUSES OF CHEST PAIN THAT ARE NOT DUE TO CORONARY ARTERY DISEASE

- Gall bladder disease
- Hiatus hernia
- Esophagitis or esophageal spasm

- Peptic ulcer
- Musculoskeletal pain
- Cervical spine disease
- Mitral valve prolapse
- Pericarditis
- Anxiety states
- Pulmonary embolus
- Dissecting aneurysm

What complications may follow a heart attack?

A whole host of complications may ensue during the course of a heart attack and the early recovery. These are shown in the accompanying table.

Table 1.2. Complications During and After a Heart Attack.

COMPLICATION	COMMENTS
Ventricular tachycardia	Very serious arrhythmias
Ventricular fibrillation (a chaotic heart rhythm)	Usually cause cardiac arrest
Heart block	Technical term for low heart rate
Heart failure	Decreased pumping strength due to muscle damage Cardiogenic shock Life-threatening decrease in pumping strength, due to severe muscle damage
Mitral regurgitation	Leaking of the mitral valve (due to weakened muscle near the mitral valve apparatus)

Embolization	Throwing-off of clots to other organs from the internal surface of the heart (the brain is especially vulnerable)
Ventricular septal defect	Hole in the heart from internal "blow-out" between right and left ventricles
Cardiac rupture	"Blow-out" of free wall of heart
Pericarditis	Irritation of heart membranes by dead muscle
Death	May be the sequel to many of the above complications

While this enumeration is daunting, please keep in mind that the vast majority of patients suffering a heart attack not only survive but also return to active lifestyles. The key is to get to the hospital as soon as possible. Many of these potential complications can be prevented or lessened by early treatment. Even the most severe complications, like internal and external cardiac rupture, can be treated by surgery or other means.

I've suffered a heart attack. How will my life change? Will I be physically handicapped by this?

We can understand your concern and fear about the future, especially if this was your first cardiac event. The fact is that most patients who suffer a heart attack will go on to lead active, productive, and, in many cases, long lives. Luckily, we are made with more heart muscle than we need. We can usually afford to lose a chunk or two without much discernible impact on lifestyle or capabilities or limitations. Yes, you will likely be on some medications. Yes, you may need an angioplasty, or even surgery. But unless your heart attack is extremely extensive, or you suffer multiple or repeated attacks, chances are that you will be able to carry on well with the activities of daily life.

2
HEART FAILURE

Case 1: The Impatient CEO.

Mr. Henning was not a happy camper. He had been waiting in the office for the surgeon (one of the authors). His pacing, his sighs, and his whispered comments to his wife all indicated his displeasure that his surgeon had not yet appeared. Mr. Henning had come up from Florida, where he had been diagnosed with end-stage heart failure. The surgeon had been detained in the operating room with a procedure that took longer than expected. Most patients are very understanding, figuring that soon they themselves might be that patient on the table who needs extra time. Not Mr. Henning. He had just recently retired as the CEO of one of the largest of the Fortune 500 companies. No one, but no one, kept him waiting. The staff in the office did their best. They sent him for coffee. They gave him patient-directed reading materials and videotapes.

When the surgeon arrived, Mr. Henning was just about fit to be tied. He insisted on being seen even before urgent messages from the morning's calls had been relayed to the surgeon.

As it turns out, Mr. Henning was already seething with anger at his cardiac circumstances. He had been healthy all his life. He had the best doctors. He followed the most stringent diets du jour. He had a personal trainer. (And, he thought, of course not voicing this aspect, he had already had a mistress or two to relieve stress throughout his life.) He had a home gym, an Olympic-sized pool with a cover for the winter months, and a one-mile running track on his property. He couldn't possibly have heart disease. It just didn't add up. It wasn't fair, in view of all he had done to maintain his health, cardiac and otherwise.

Yet, for months now, he had become more and more short of breath. At first, he found he had to cut out his jogging. Later, he could no longer do his weights. Later still, he couldn't walk to the mailbox (albeit down the eighth of a mile driveway). Most recently, he had been awakened from sleep, unable to breathe. Even the fresh nighttime air had not been sufficient, and he had made several nocturnal trips to the emergency room. His personal physician was waiting for him each time. Each time, a water drug, Lasix, had been administered via IV, producing prompt improvement. He must have passed a gallon of urine each night, after the Lasix, Mr. Henning recalled.

The requisite tests had been done by his Florida physician. The chest X-ray had shown severe congestive heart failure, with water in the lungs and a large heart. The EKG had been normal, with no evidence of heart attack damage. The echocardiogram had shown a large and very weak heart, with enlargement and poor contraction of both the left and right sides of the heart. A catheterization had shown that all the arteries were clear—this was not arteriosclerosis.

It had been a virus, the Florida cardiologist had told Mr. Henning and his wife. In 999 of 1,000 patients, the virus would have produced a simple cold. In Mr. Henning, it had chosen to attack his heart muscle, inflicting heavy damage. As no improvement had been realized, the cardiologist had indicated that the condition was likely irreversible. "End-stage heart failure," he had been told. The outlook was not good.

Mr. Henning was pissed. Fate had no right to do this to him. Not at the age of seventy-one, when he had just retired from a lifetime of fourteen-hour days, ready to enjoy the considerable fruits of his labors. It was not fair. He could not accept it. He would not accept it. "What can be done? Who is the best? Can't they operate? Where can I go to be seen?" These were Mr. Henning's questions—or, more accurately, his commands—to his capable local physicians. They had better find something to be done, or they would be in deep trouble, his manner and his words conveyed.

So, he wound up in the surgeon's office—upset at his condition—and seething at being kept waiting.

The surgeon apologized for the delay and promised his fullest attention and the most thorough consultation.

The exam was consistent with heart failure. The pulse was rapid. There was a heart murmur, indicating that the mitral valve was leaking, due to the excess strain on the heart. There were crackles audible in the lungs, indicating continued presence of excess fluid. His ankles were swollen. Except for his heart failure, Mr. Henning was a picture of health. And his mind, though his attitude was caustic, was as sharp as any mind in an individual of any age.

The answers were clear. The surgeon delivered the information as patiently and gently as possible. Mr. Henning indeed was suffering from advanced heart failure, end-stage, in fact. It would not improve. It would just worsen. And, Mr. Henning was too old—a severe frown appeared on Henning's face at those words—for either a heart transplant or an artificial heart. Medical treatment—with drugs—was the only option.

He would not and could not accept that. Those were Henning's words as he and his entourage of chauffeurs, bodyguards, and various assistants stormed out the door of the surgeon's office.

How common is heart failure?

Heart failure is the one cardiac illness that is actually becoming more widespread at the present time. Other cardiac diseases are coming under control, as the result of improved medications and preventive treatments. Not so heart failure.

About three million Americans currently suffer from heart failure. Over four hundred thousand new patients are diagnosed as suffering from heart failure each year.

Why should heart failure be increasing? In large part, the increase in heart failure is a reflection of medical improvements in care of initial cardiac emergencies.

For example, patients who suffered cardiac arrest in earlier decades often did not survive. Now, with cardiopulmonary resuscitation techniques familiar to a broad spectrum of the general population, many victims of cardiac arrest are successfully resuscitated. These patients, although they survive, often have suffered severe cardiac damage and eventually develop overt heart failure. Likewise, in the past, patients who arrived at the hospital with a massive heart attack tended not to live for very long. Now, with cardiac support by drugs and devices, thrombolytic medications, and other advances, patients with a large heart attack often survive the initial episode; years thereafter, they often manifest heart failure.

The advent of the implantable cardioverter defibrillator—one of the devices mentioned above—now effectively prevents the arrhythmic deaths that often took patients' lives in the past. These patients now survive, often going on to develop heart failure.

In sum, by effectively combating early cardiac death from devastating acute events, medical science is creating a large group of patients who survive but have suffered so much cardiac damage that the pumping strength of the heart is severely depressed. These patients develop the manifestations of heart failure.

How do you grade the severity of heart failure?

A precise scale for grading the severity of heart failure has been used by heart specialists for many decades. It is called the New York Heart Association grading system, and it assigns grades by roman numerals, from I to IV, as severity increases.

Grade I patients have no excess shortness of breath regardless of intensity of exertion. Grade II patients experience shortness of breath with moderate exertion, like walking up a steep hill. Grade III patients experience shortness of breath with only mild exertion, like performing housework. Grade IV patients are short of breath at rest; this is a very disturbing situation that is usually very frightening and poorly tolerated.

My doctor told me I have a very large heart. Isn't bigger better?

In some things in life, bigger may be better, but not as far as the size of your heart is concerned. Your heart is best off the size that it was before you got heart disease. The problem with heart failure is that your heart gets bigger and bigger. This occurs for two reasons. First, your body holds on to fluid, so that the heart becomes fuller and stretches. Second, as it weakens, your heart doesn't contract as strongly. By getting bigger, your heart gets a little more blood propelled forward with each heartbeat than it would at its normal size. The process of enlargement, unfortunately, represents a vicious cycle. The heart is hurt by getting bigger, and thus becomes bigger still because it is hurt more. This is diagrammed schematically in the Figure 2.1.

Some initial insult leads to a weakening of the heart. This can be a heart attack—probably the most common cause—an infection, or a leaky valve could be the inciting event. Over the course of time, cumulative insults weaken the heart more and more, leading to progressively more severe cardiac enlargement. In many cases, the outcome, without optimal treatment, can be fatal. Figure 2.2 shows the process of progressive heart failure from cumulative insults.

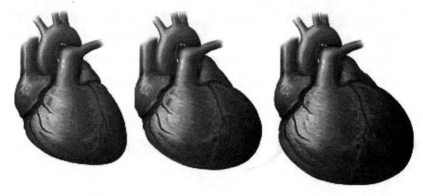

The Progression of Heart Failure

Figure 2.1. Progression of heart failure. Courtesy of Acorn Cardiovascular.

What is the cause of shortness of breath (dyspnea) in patients with cardiac disease?

The medical term dyspnea refers to the subjective sensation of shortness of breath, an awareness of the act of breathing. Most of the time, breathing is an automatic act that we do not have to think about. Cardiac dyspnea generally occurs when the heart's pumping action has become weakened. At times it may be due to a narrowing in the mitral or aortic valve, which causes obstruction to the free

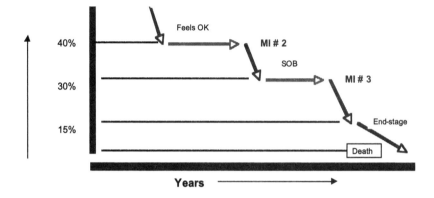

MI = Myocardial infarction (heart attack)
SOB = Short of breath

A typical pattern of repeated heart attacks over many years. Note that the patient feels OK after the first heart attack. His ejection fraction (EF) may drop from a normal 55% to about 40%. With the second heart attack, as his EF falls to 30%, he becomes short of breath. With the third heart attack, with his EF now down to 15%, he is in serious trouble; he may be in and out of the hospital, often on powerful IV drugs. Death may ensue.

Please note that this scenario is selected as a representative example. None of these numbers is absolute. Patients may respond variably to heart attacks and different levels of EF.

Figure 2.2. Cumulative insults resulting in eventual heart failure.

Case 2. Breathing Becomes Short for the Track Star.

David was seventeen, a high school senior in a small rural town in Connecticut.

The first sign of trouble was that he stopped winning his cross-country meets. He had been the team's star. Between his natural talent and his concerted training, he was a force to be reckoned with in Connecticut track and field. That's why he didn't understand what was happening. He was training just as hard—harder even—and putting in a 200 percent effort during the meets, but he wasn't winning anymore.

After a few weeks, he couldn't finish the runs at all. In another week, he had to stop going to practice. He and his parents thought he had just burned out after years of extreme effort at his chosen sport.

Then, one night, he awoke

during the night, unable to breathe. He had to go to an open window, just to catch his breath.

In our emergency room, there were dramatic findings that we communicated to the incredulous patient and his anxious family. The cause of David's shortness of breath was heart failure. There was no doubt about it. The chest X-ray showed that this otherwise healthy young man had lungs full of fluid. Also, the heart was dramatically enlarged. This had not happened overnight, we explained. These changes needed a minimum of weeks to months to occur.

The diagnosis, we explained, was idiopathic cardiomyopathy, which means advanced weakness of the heart without an apparent cause. Once in a blue moon, we told the family, an ordinary cold, instead of producing just some sniffles, a fever, and a sore throat, can actually infect the heart muscle, leading to severe damage to the heart cells themselves.

Out of millions of viruses and colds, only a few could cause such a problem.

David stayed in the hospital, and we started various heart failure treatments. When he went home, we had already listed him for heart transplantation. Our hope was that a heart would become available for David before his heart deteriorated any further.

It turns out that David had an uncle who had died in his twenties of a similar problem. We cardiologists had thought for many years that having a virus affect the heart was just a fluke. In recent years, we had noticed, these viral cardiomyopathies clustered in families. David, it appeared, proved the rule. The inciting virus is clearly the effect of environmental factors, but the predisposition to have the virus attack the heart was genetic. This disease served for medical science as another example of environment and heredity interacting in ways we had not previously understood.

flow of blood through the heart into the major blood vessels. Whatever the cause, shortness of breath occurs because blood and fluids
begin to back up behind the heart. This increases the pressure in the
pulmonary veins, ultimately resulting in a leaking of fluid from the
bloodstream into the air sacs in the lungs. The leaking of fluid into
the air sacs of the lungs makes the lungs stiffer and increases the
work of breathing. This represents essentially an internal
"drowning" of the lungs. The awareness that it is harder to breathe
is the symptom of dyspnea.

When it is severe, dyspnea of cardiac origin is called *pulmonary
edema.* This feels like drowning from fluid in one's own lungs. The
patients are uncomfortable, struggling, and frightened. The accompanying figure conveys the typical appearance of a patient suffering
from pulmonary edema.

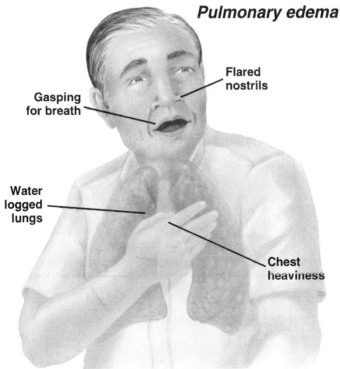

Figure 2.3. Pulmonary edema.

I used to be able to walk up three flights of stairs without stopping. Now I have to wait at the first landing to catch my breath. Does this mean I have heart disease?

Not all dyspnea is due to cardiac problems. Dyspnea may be due to a pulmonary problem, even though the heart may be normal. Shortness of breath as a result of lung disease stems from narrowing or stiffening of the airways, which makes it difficult to get air in and out of the lungs, or from destruction of the lungs as a result of smoking. People with asthma or emphysema often experience dyspnea due to pulmonary causes. (Some extremely sedentary individuals can also impair their lung function by virtue of inactivity.) Distinguishing between cardiac dyspnea and pulmonary dyspnea is not always simple. Generally, people with pulmonary dyspnea, whose lungs have lost their suppleness over a long period of time, tend to breathe more slowly and deeply, especially in moving air out of the lungs. Patients with cardiac dyspnea tend to move air in and out of the lungs in short, rapid, shallow breaths. In answer to your question, shortness of breath can be cardiac or pulmonary in origin. Your physician should be able to distinguish between the two by appropriate testing.

At the end of the day, my ankles often swell. Is this a sign of heart disease?

Ankle swelling is called edema. It is a common finding in patients with heart disease but may be present for a variety of other reasons, none of which are related to heart disease. If edema results from heart disease, it is because of a buildup of pressure behind the right heart. This elevated pressure causes an increase of pressure in the veins leading to the right heart, virtually squeezing fluid through the spaces between the cells that make up the walls of the small veins. The result is that fluid accumulates in the tissue surrounding the veins, especially in the lower legs. It is gravity that pulls the fluid to that location. Edema usually means that salt and water are being retained as well. The accompanying figure illustrates characteristics of edema.

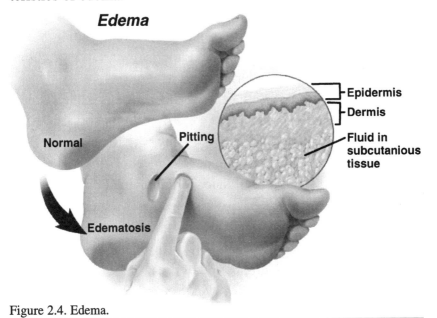

Figure 2.4. Edema.

There are a number of noncardiac reasons for ankle swelling. After heart disease, the second major cause of edema is kidney disease. In such a circumstance, the kidney is not getting rid of salt and water adequately, thus allowing fluid to build up in the body.

Edema may also be caused by liver disease. Albumin, which is made by the liver, is a vital protein in the blood that keeps fluid from escaping from the blood vessels into the surrounding tissues. Albumin is normally like a sponge, keeping fluid within the blood vessels. Liver diseases, such as cirrhosis, caused by alcoholism, may adversely affect the production of albumin and thus cause edema.

Certain medications, particularly calcium channel blockers used to treat high blood pressure, may cause ankle swelling. Part of their action is to dilate the small arteries and veins in the body, and this may lead to leaking of fluid into the surrounding tissue. Since most individuals are in the upright position for most of the day, the fluid tends to accumulate in the most dependent parts, the legs. It is not uncommon for edema to disappear overnight, during which time the individual has been supine. Fluid may start to re-accumulate when the person is up during the day.

Edema may also be a sign of local abnormalities in the veins of the lower extremities, especially if varicose veins are present. Also, if the lymphatic drainage system is in any way impaired (as from growths or tumors), there may be development of edema.

Finally, edema may occur under certain normal circumstances, as on a hot day when you have consumed much water in conjunction with salty foods. Edema is also normal during the late stages of pregnancy and is not uncommon in travelers who have been seated in airplanes for a long period of time.

The appearance of edema, however, should prompt a visit to a physician so that the above possibilities can be sorted out.

I find myself fatigued by early evening. What causes fatigue?

The cause of fatigue can be very elusive. Fatigue may be the result of a variety of physical diseases, but it may also be a symptom of depression. At times, a patient may be depressed because he has a physical disease. If fatigue is due solely to heart disease, the patient usually feels refreshed upon waking in the morning and then gets fatigued as the day wears on. In a patient whose fatigue is due to depression, fatigue is usually present upon rising and persists all day long. The likely reason why patients with heart disease complain of fatigue has to do with the heart not pumping blood adequately to the tissues of the body.

It must be recognized, however, that certain drugs, particularly beta-blockers, may cause fatigue. Such medications slow the heart rate and decrease cardiac output in addition to treating hypertension. In addition to the cardiac effects of beta-blockers, these medications may lead to fatigue secondary to their effect on the brain.

Other physical causes of fatigue include anemia, hypothyroidism, chronic lung disease, and diabetes.

Also, it must be remembered that individuals who wake early in the morning may feel fatigued toward the end of the day simply because they would have been awake by that time for many hours.

Finally, we must remember that age plays a role as well. None of us has the same energy that we had when we were younger.

ARRHYTHMIAS

Case 1: Shocking Events at the Local Bar.

Jeff was a big man, tall as a basketball player, and strong and wide as a football player. He was sixty-two. He still thought of himself as a tough guy. He had a checkered past, having had, during his life, a run-in or two with the law.

Fifteen years ago, he had the big one. He suffered a massive, transmural anterior wall myocardial infarction. What those words mean, one by one, is: a very large, through-and-through heart attack affecting the front wall of the heart.

His doctor had told him that the dead anterior wall of his heart had stretched, becoming thin like an orange peel, forming the bulge known as a left ventric-ular aneurysm—an aneurysm of the main pumping chamber of the heart.

Sure, he got short of breath every now and then, mainly when carrying heavy loads at the shipping station, where he was supervisor. Also, he admitted to himself that carrying the extra forty pounds around his middle was not doing any good for his exercise capacity.

But as far as he was concerned, that so-called aneurysm was not bothering him at all. He couldn't feel it; he wasn't even aware of its presence.

Until last night. At the pool hall, he was about to go for a ricochet shot into the corner pocket (with ten dollars at stake), when he suddenly went pale and fell right over onto the pool table.

As the crowd responded to the commotion, two men took immediate action. One was a fireman, the other a policeman. They lifted the whale of a man onto the pool table, felt for his pulse—nondetectable—and immediately started CPR. Their professions required that they be skilled in this life-saving technique.

Bill, the policeman, compressed the breast—hard, as required—at eighty times per minute. Eric, the fireman, breathed for the collapsed man, mouth-to-mouth, as no mechanical breathing equipment was available.

They could tell that Jeff had suffered a full-blown cardiac arrest. Although they were both off-duty, as far as they were concerned, it had happened "on their watch," and they were determined to bring Jeff through.

Jeff had stirred once or twice as the policeman and the fireman did their CPR, indicating that their efforts were providing some blood to the stricken man's brain.

When the paramedics arrived, they put the paddles of the defibrillator immediately onto Jeff's chest, after ripping off his shirt. The repetitive, wavelike pattern indicated that Jeff was in ventricular tachycardia—one of the worst cardiac rhythms a person could have, and one that was not able to sustain forward output from the heart. Were it not for the CPR, Jeff's brain and other organs would not have been receiving any oxygen. But, fortunately, the fireman and the policeman had been there and had acted quickly.

The paramedics immediately delivered an electrical shock—an electrical defibrillation, as it is called. Jeff's arms and legs went into spasms as he lay on the pool table, involuntary signs that the electrical energy had reached his body.

Little by little, a feeble "beep, beep" was heard to emanate from the EKG machine, slowly at first, then louder and faster. Lo and behold, Jeff regained consciousness. His instinctive reaction, based on many a barroom brawl, was to punch the guy who had decked him. Jeff's powerful fist swung around, more threatening than it was coordinated.

But Jeff was after the wrong opponent. No one in the bar had been responsible. It was that aneurysm—the one he couldn't tell was there—that had reared its ugly head after fifteen years of dormancy. The aneurysm had decked the big man.

As studies in the hospital would show, the ventricular tachycardia was originating in the scarred wall of the left ventricular aneurysm, and cardiac arrest would happen again if appropriate measures were not taken.

What is an arrhythmia?

An arrhythmia is any abnormality of the basic heartbeat. The abnormality can involve the *rate* of the heart or the *rhythm* of the heartbeat. In a case of arrhythmia, it is as if the tempo or syncopation of the normal symphony of your heart has been disturbed.

Normally, the heart beats between sixty and one hundred times per minute. A heart rate of less than sixty is called a sinus bradycardia (*brady* means "slow" in Greek), and a heart rate greater than one hundred is called a sinus tachycardia (*tachy* means "fast" in Greek). The term *sinus* is good. The sinus is the normal area in the upper chamber of your heart where the heartbeat *should* originate. If the rhythm is initiated at a different site, the term *sinus* can no longer be applied, signifying a deviation from the norm.

A tachycardia that arises in the upper chamber, the atrium, is called an atrial tachycardia or atrial flutter. If the atrium is disorganized and does not initiate a regular rhythm, then the arrhythmia is likely the chaotic rhythm called atrial fibrillation. The above rhythm disturbances are generally not life-threatening.

If the tachycardia is initiated in the lower chamber, the ventricle, then the rhythm is a dangerous one. Ventricular tachycardia is often a sign of severe underlying structural disease and is a life-threatening rhythm disturbance. It signifies that the lower chambers have developed a rapid rate of their own, essentially like a runaway train. Ventricular fibrillation is the most dangerous rhythm disturbance and will lead to death if it persists for even a few minutes. In ventricular fibrillation, the heart muscle simply quivers, not even generating a single organized heartbeat.

You can get a sense of the aberrations from a normal sinus rhythm in the tracings presented in figure 3.1. The orderly, coordinated pattern seen in the top tracing can be replaced by the disorderly, extremely rapid tracings seen in the other panels.

Very slow heart rates that do not arise in the sinus node are generally due to a condition termed heart block. In this condition, the atrium and ventricles lose their electrical connection and beat separately and independently. The intrinsic beat of the ventricle is usually slower than normal and hence the heart rate is most often less than sixty beats per minute.

I feel that my heart skips. Does this mean I have heart disease?

Ordinarily people are unaware of their heartbeat. This is fortunate, as the heart of an average person beats five hundred thousand times per week. Patients describe an irregular heartbeat in a variety of ways. It is sometimes perceived as a skip, but may also be described as a fluttering in the chest—like a bird beating its wings

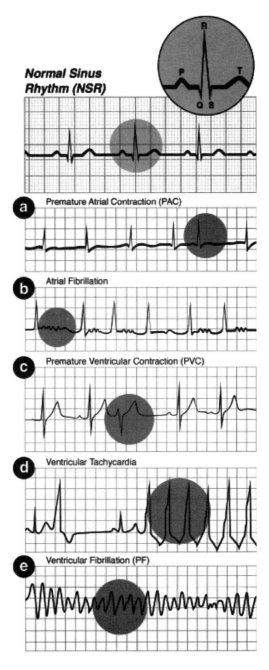

Figure 3.1. Common arrhythmias.

or as a thumping, flip-flopping, or pounding in the chest or neck, or even as a tickle in the throat region. The most common form of palpitation is not due to heart disease but may simply be a heightened awareness of the heartbeat because of anxiety or tension.

Palpitations are most often due to a premature atrial or ventricular beat. The heart normally beats quite regularly, with each beat occurring at the same interval as the previous one. On occasion, an extra beat will occur prematurely and the regularity of the rhythm will be disturbed. This premature beat will be followed by a heavy beat, as if the heart is trying to get caught up. This will be felt as an extra beat.

Even in the absence of any heart disease, palpitations may be brought on by caffeine-containing beverages (coffee, tea, sodas), smoking, alcohol, emotions, or some prescription drugs used to treat asthma or other lung disorders.

Although most cardiac skips or arrhythmias are not serious, they should be brought to the attention of a physician.

How does a physician go about diagnosing a patient with palpitations?

A patient's history is sometimes a clue to the nature of an abnormal heart rhythm. Sudden onset or sudden cessation, regularity or irregularity, rapid or slow, these are helpful clues. At times a simple test, the electrocardiogram (EKG), will tell the story. But the electrocardiogram records less than one minute of the heart's action, and there are 1,440 minutes in a day. If the arrhythmia is present while the electrocardiogram is being taken, often no other investigation is necessary. The next step in unraveling the symptom is a test using a Holter monitor. This test requires the patient to wear a device that records all of the heartbeats over a twenty-four-hour period. Three or four small EKG pads are placed over the chest, and the data are sent to a tape recorder worn by the patient. The patient makes a written record of the time of occurrence of any symptoms. The time of these symptoms can then be correlated with what was happening with the heart's rhythm. Sometimes this pinpoints the difficulty, but often the patient may feel there is a symptom even though the tape shows perfectly normal heart rate and rhythm.

If the EKG and Holter monitor are not helpful, then the patient may be given an event recorder. This is a device that the patient uses for about a month. There is a continuous tape loop that erases itself after a built-in delay. If the patient senses a symptom, the electrocardiogram can be transmitted telephonically and recorded at the monitoring center. Since arrhythmias are often random, intermittent, and infrequent, the event recorder is often helpful in identifying the underlying abnormal heart rhythm causing the symptoms.

Finally, the most sophisticated technique available for identifying an arrhythmia is called EP, or electrophysiologic testing. This is a technique in which a catheter is placed in the atrium or ventricle and electrical stimulation is given to the heart. The goal of this procedure is to identify the type of arrhythmia present by provoking the abnormal rhythm electrically. Then the most effective therapy, either with drugs or by catheter or even by surgery, can be performed for the patient.

My doctor said I would need an EP test. What exactly is that?

An EP test, or electrophysiological test, delivers electrical stimuli via a catheter threaded into your heart. The purpose of the test is to see if electrical stimuli can cause your heart to enter an abnormal rhythm, such as ventricular tachycardia or ventricular fibrillation.

Your doctor would not be ordering this test unless it was important. Chances are that you have had such an arrhythmia or one of its precursors before. Alternatively, if you have suffered a major heart attack and have severely depressed ejection fraction (low pumping strength of your heart), your doctor may feel that you are at risk for arrhythmia in the future.

The EP test is highly effective in predicting your susceptibility to future serious arrhythmic events. If the test is negative—your heart cannot be tickled electrically into a serious arrhythmia—your outlook is very good. If, on the other hand, your arrhythmia is easily induced during the EP test, chances are very high that you will have a serious arrhythmia during your daily activities. In such a case, some treatment may be recommended.

This EP test sounds very dangerous. Why would I want someone to deliberately put me into ventricular tachycardia?

Believe it or not, this type of test is very safe. Patients rarely have major adverse consequences during or after such testing. Yes, you may—and probably will—need to be defibrillated during the course of this test, but, in this setting, that is routine. The doctors who do this test are specially trained and skilled at recognition and management of these serious rhythm abnormalities, and the information will be of great importance for your future safety. Also, you will be sedated appropriately, and chances are you will not have discomfort or even a recollection of the events of the test itself.

What causes slow heart rate?

In many cases, slow heart rate is caused by the wear and tear of aging. The spot of tissue in the right atrium that normally initiates

Case 2: It's My Head That Hurts, Not My Heart.

We were called to the emergency room to see a Mr. Voytek. He was eighty-five years old, we had been told. He was working in his garden when he suddenly dropped to the ground, hitting his head on a rock, which lacerated his scalp.

Why were they calling the cardiac team? Because this was a classic case of a drop attack. The patient had literally "dropped" to the ground. This was the classic textbook scenario for loss of consciousness from sudden cessation of cardiac output. Often, a very low heart rate was the root cause, and it certainly appeared to be the cause here.

Mr. Voytek's terrified eighty-one-year-old wife of fifty-nine years had called 911, which was the right thing to do. Mr. Voytek was drifting in and out of consciousness when the paramedics arrived, rubbing the bleeding gash on his scalp when he was conscious.

The senior paramedic had felt Mr. Voytek's neck for his pulse. "Extreme brady-cardia" is what she had called out to her colleagues, meaning seriously slow heart rate. She counted out a pulse rate of thirty-five beats per minute, hardly enough for even a younger person to sustain adequate forward output from the heart and maintain consciousness.

They had hurried Mr. Voytek into the ambulance and hooked him up to the EKG, revealing what they called "complete heart block," or an interruption of the conduction of electrical impulses between the upper cardiac chambers, where the electrical activity of the heart originates, and the lower cardiac chambers, which actually do most of the pumping.

The paramedics had spoken to our ER doctors and, upon their approval (based on the EKG tracing that had been telemetered while the ambulance was in transit) atropine had been administered. Atropine is a powerful heart rate t-raising medication. Mr. Voytek had remained conscious from that time on. The paramedics had also started an IV and administered some salt solution, which helped to improve his cardiac output.

What we found in the ER was an elderly man totally unaware of what had transpired and why his head hurt so much. He couldn't understand why everyone was making such a big deal over his heart, when it was his head that hurt.

We were able to confirm that Mr. Voytek was in complete heart block. The eighty-five-year-old's "electrical wires" inside his heart had finally given way, and the function of his heart had been suddenly, acutely—and rudely, from his perspective—interrupted. Now, however, his body had adapted a bit; nature, in her unbounded wisdom, had encouraged the lower chambers to generate their own heartbeat. It would never be as good as the one from above—it was now generating fifty-three beats instead of the normal seventy-two—but it was sufficient for the time being.

We recommended to Mr. Voytek that we place a permanent pacemaker in his heart. This would monitor his heartbeat and ensure that it never fell low again—absolutely, positively preventing any further drop attacks due to inadequate heart rate.

Mr. Voytek agreed, reluctantly, concerned that we were mistaken in treating his heart when, from his point of view, the problem was still located at the throbbing wound over his right temple.

the heartbeat may become "tired" with age and fail in its function. The electrical "wires," which normally transmit the electrical impulse throughout the heart muscle, may become dysfunctional with age. In fact, these "wires" are actually made of nerve cells, which degenerate with aging.

In other cases, a heart attack may cause the death of important nerve cells, just as it affects the heart muscle itself. In such a case, a slow heart rate results.

Rarely, heart block may be caused by an internal infection within the heart. Lyme disease, rampant in the northeast United States, is one such potential cause of heart block, even among young individuals.

What is meant by the conduction system of the heart?

The conduction system of the heart is electrical in nature. A specialized tissue called the sinus node initiates the signal that triggers a heartbeat. The electrical wave spreads over the atria to a second specialized tissue called the atrioventricular node. From there the conduction wave enters the ventricles through channels called the left- and right-bundle branches. As the electrical wave activates the ventricular muscle, the ventricles contract, ejecting blood respectively into the lungs from the right ventricle and into the aorta from the left ventricle. Over the course of a lifetime, the electrical system activates the heart over two billion times. It is a remarkable system in that even a four- or five-second failure may lead to a state where unconsciousness will occur.

It is when the conduction system starts to falter, usually after many decades of continuous activity, that a cardiac pacemaker may be required.

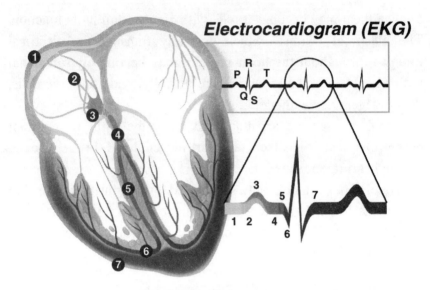

Figure 3.2. An electrocardiogram showing the conducting system of the heart. The fine biological "wires" conduct the heartbeat in sequence from the upper to the lower chambers of the heart.

I recently fainted while I was exerting myself. What might have caused it?

The medical word for fainting is *syncope*. Fainting usually results after the brain has been deprived of oxygen and blood for about ten seconds. The general causes of fainting include cardiac problems, diseases of the brain, and a variety of abnormalities of the arteries and veins that secondarily cause inadequate blood flow to the brain.

Fainting that occurs during exercise or directly thereafter is often cardiac in origin. It may be due to a ventricular arrhythmia precipitated by inadequate coronary blood flow during exercise. It may also reflect one of two conditions representing obstruction to the flow of blood as it leaves the heart. These may be due to valvular narrowing, called *aortic valve stenosis*, or a muscular narrowing, called *hypertrophic cardiomyopathy*, which also causes obstruction.

Also, fainting may occur due to complete heart block where the rate of the heart cannot increase enough to keep the brain oxygenated. At times, very rapid heart rates may lead to syncope, as the heart does not have sufficient time between beats to fill in preparation for the next ejection.

Syncope can also be due to an obstruction in the blood vessels in the neck that carry blood and oxygen to the brain. The carotid arteries serve as conduits for blood and oxygen to the brain. Severe narrowing may limit blood flow through arteries to the brain.

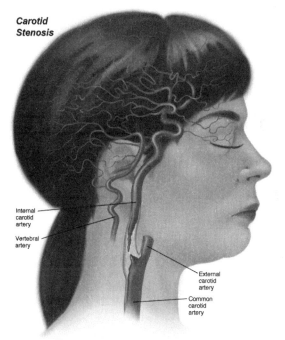

Figure 3.3. Schematic of brain affected by carotid artery stenosis.

At times, fainting may be mediated through the nervous system. The vagus nerve, when stimulated, slows the heart rate. In certain individuals, intense emotion may activate the vagus, leading to profound slowing of the heart rate and fainting. The classic "Victorian faint" is of such a variety. Fainting at the sight of blood is probably another example.

Finally, there exists a collection of nerves within the neck called the carotid sinus. In the presence of an overactive carotid sinus, the vagus nerve can be activated. Turning the head in one or another direction or bending the neck may activate the carotid sinus and lead to fainting.

Fortunately, these types of fainting are usually transient—and of short enough duration that brain cells do not die, so that there is no permanent damage.

Causes of Fainting

- Slow heart rate
- Carotid artery narrowing
- Cardiac arrhythmias
- Aortic valve stenosis
- During urination (micturition syncope)
- Hypertrophic obstructive cardiomyopathy (physical obstruction of outflow of heart due to a muscle-bound state below the aortic valve)
- After cough (cough syncope)
- Low blood pressure
- Epilepsy
- Vasovagal syncope ("Victorian swoon"; anxiety, fright)
- Allergic reaction (bee sting, or other)
- Dehydration

Last year I had a TIA. This year I fainted. Are these events related?

A TIA—the medical abbreviation for transient ischemic attack— is a temporary deprivation of the blood supply to the brain.

The two events you describe are probably related. Carotid

artery stenoses are composed of plaques that narrow the channel within the carotid artery. The narrowing may lead to a TIA in one or two ways. First, it may limit blood flow for a sufficient period to cause neurologic symptoms. Second, it may cause neurologic symptoms after particulate matter—either a small blood clot (thrombus) or a cholesterol embolus (traveling particle)—breaks free and lodges in a cerebral blood vessel. The two events are not identical, but they are related, and each can lead to an episode of fainting.

I recently fainted while standing at the urinal. Does this mean I have a heart problem?

Not necessarily. There is a particular type of fainting that is precipitated by urination, most often when the individual strains while standing up. The sensation of a full bladder, in conjunction with strain, activates the vagus nerve, thereby slowing the heart rate and simultaneously decreasing the return of blood from the lower extremities. These two effects in concert may lead to inadequate cerebral blood flow and a fainting episode. If this occurs repeatedly, you need to see your doctor for evaluation and treatment.

What causes atrial fibrillation?

In some cases, we can identify specific causes for atrial fibrillation. For example, the strain of a blocked mitral valve, called *mitral stenosis*, can cause the left atrium to struggle, enlarge, and lapse into atrial fibrillation.

In most cases, however, atrial fibrillation is just due to aging and wear and tear on the heart. In fact, up to 15 percent of patients over the age of eighty have had atrial fibrillation at some point.

Case 3: The Doctor's Mom and Her Fluttering Heart.

The atrial fibrillation was driving her mother crazy, Dr. Martha Matthews was telling one of the authors on the phone. Martha was a doctor, an ophthalmologist, but she admitted to knowing almost nothing about the heart. That's about as much as I know about the eye, the author thought to himself.

Mom was seventy-eight. She had been in very good health. Two months ago, she had developed atrial fibrillation, an arrhythmia, or abnormal heart rhythm, to which the elderly are especially prone. With this abnormal rhythm, the upper chambers of the heart contract at a very rapid rate (often up to 180 beats per minute or more) and in a very irregular pattern. That was exactly why Mom Matthews felt the rapid fluttering, or palpitations, in her chest. She didn't like it one bit. It just didn't feel right. It felt dangerous. It felt like she should do something—

move, or cough, or drink some water—but nothing made it feel better.

Dr. Matthews explained that her mother's energy was down dramatically since the atrial fibrillation had come on. That was not surprising, as the loss of slow, regular contractions of the upper chambers robbed the heart of 15 to 20 percent of its output.

And the medications were a great burden to Mom Matthews, her daughter explained. There were the antiarrhythmics, the drugs aimed at restoring a normal pattern of heartbeat. Then, there were the blocking drugs, the ones meant to bring the heart rate down from the stratosphere. And, above all, those blood thinners were troublesome. The family doctor had explained that, with the atrial fibrillation, Mrs. Matthews was at risk for developing clots in the heart, clots that could travel to the brain and cause a stroke.

Stroke was a word Mrs. Matthews had not wanted to hear. She had seen too many of her elderly friends go down that path.

So, Dr. Matthews explained, Mom liked nothing about this new atrial fibrillation. Wasn't there something we could do about it? Couldn't we set it right again—with meds or electrical paddles, or something?

A visit was scheduled, and we looked forward to meeting Mrs. Matthews and fine-tuning her cardiac care.

Will my atrial fibrillation be permanent?

In some cases, drugs or electrical conversion may restore a sustained normal rhythm. In many cases, unfortunately, the atrial fibrillation will be permanent. In such cases, controlling the overall heart rate with drugs diminishes the subjective sensations felt by the patient. The rhythm is still technically atrial fibrillation, but with the racing heart rate now controlled, the patient is not as aware of the aberration. Many elderly patients cease to be aware of the arrhythmia entirely, essentially becoming "used to it."

I have heard that atrial fibrillation can be eliminated by a procedure. Is this true?

There are indeed multiple procedures performed in the catheterization laboratory and in the operating room that are aimed at eliminating atrial fibrillation.

A remarkable heart surgeon, Dr. James Cox, formerly of Washington University in St. Louis, devoted his career to the study of arrhythmias, including atrial fibrillation. Together with his brilliant colleagues, he elucidated the electrical pathways within the atria, or upper chambers of the heart, that permit atrial fibrillation to be sustained. Based on these intensive investigations, he devised a surgical procedure to prevent atrial fibrillation.[1] This procedure involved dividing the atria into smaller compartments and channels so that atrial fibrillation could no longer be maintained. The development of this procedure represents one of the most significant present-day accomplishments in cardiology.

Dr. Cox's procedure became known as the Maze procedure because the smaller channels and compartments resembled a maze that the electrical signals of the heart needed to traverse. The Maze procedure was formidable surgically, requiring multiple incisions in the atrial chambers as well as freezing certain critical spots within the atria. The procedure was adopted with moderate enthusiasm, but it was such a complex, time-consuming operation that it was never applied widely in everyday practice. At institutions where it was practiced, the procedure was highly effective in preventing atrial fibrillation permanently.

Currently, there is great enthusiasm for trying to re-create the Maze operation with new equipment that electrically "fries" trenches in the atrial tissue, thus avoiding the need for time-consuming incisions. These operations, called Maze operations, fall far short of Dr. Cox's true intention. These procedures are perhaps better termed *partial* or *mini*-Maze procedures, as none re-creates the original operation fully. The advantage is that these procedures are quick and can often be performed as an adjunct to other open heart surgery. These procedures can even be performed minimally invasively, through small chest incisions, with a relatively short hospital stay.

The effectiveness of these mini-Maze procedures is as yet unclear. Many patients continue to have atrial fibrillation, to need drugs, and to undergo periodic electrical cardioversions. If you would like to learn more about these procedures, discuss the matter fully with your cardiologist and your cardiothoracic surgeon.

Not surprisingly, efforts are even under way to partially re-create the Maze operation by a catheter technique in the catheterization laboratory without any incision at all. This is called ablation therapy for atrial fibrillation. These procedures are even less invasive than the mini-Maze surgical procedures. Like the mini-Maze, their effectiveness is still in question, with some good results but many recurrences. You should explore the benefits and risks fully with your cardiologist. The jury is still out on this topic.

I have heard about a new device that can be placed inside the heart to prevent a stroke in a patient with atrial fibrillation. Tell me about this.

There is indeed a new device, called the WATCHMAN, now entering clinical trials.[2] See figure 3.4.

WATCHMAN® LAA System

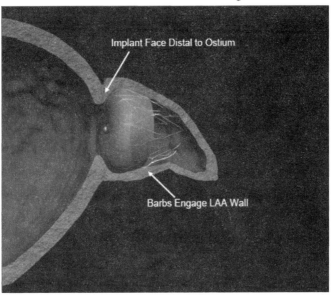

Figure 3.4. The WATCHMAN device, intended to prevent clots from forming in and dislodging from the left atrial appendage in patients with atrial fibrillation. The left atrial appendage is the blind pouch portion of the left atrium. This is where clots start. The umbrellalike WATCHMAN device obliterates the connection of the left atrial appendage to the body of the left atrium, thus preventing clots from reaching the circulation. Courtesy of Atritech.

In atrial fibrillation, the atrial chambers of the heart, the upper chambers, do not beat effectively. Rather, they quiver. For this reason, blood is not propelled as effectively as it should be. So, clots can form. These clots almost always originate from a blind pouch that connects with the main chamber of the left atrium. This blind pouch is called the *atrial appendage*, because it looks very much like your body's appendix (in your belly).

It is well known that clots formed from atrial fibrillation always originate in the atrial appendage. This is because blood is very stagnant in that blind pouch, so patients without a coordinated heartbeat of the upper chambers, that is, patients with atrial fibrillation, are susceptible to this problem.

At surgery, we often excise this atrial appendage in patients with atrial fibrillation. As with your body's appendix, removal of the heart's appendix causes no harm. In fact, removal of the heart's appendix, in patients with atrial fibrillation, provides excellent protection from clots and stroke. The excision of the atrial appendage is usually done in conjunction with another cardiac procedure; we "are already there," so to speak, so we take out the atrial appendage as well. Sometimes, we operate expressly for this purpose, although not very often. Cardiologists and patients are not usually eager to have a surgical procedure for this sole purpose.

The WATCHMAN device is intended to mimic the effectiveness of surgical excision of the left atrial appendage. The device is placed by catheter, in the catheterization laboratory. It resides in the atrial appendage, closing off that blind pouch like a curtain. We will look forward to results from the early clinical trials. This device holds some promise.

Chapter 4

VALVULAR HEART DISEASE

Case 1: The Mystery Patient with a Leaking Mitral Valve.

Hey, John! Clark was on the phone. He was calling about a patient. Dr. Elefteriades was very pleased to hear from his former coresident. They had cut their teeth together in the days when chief residents were given extreme responsibility, probably more than their experience justified. Their mentors knew they would grow into it. Clark and John had supported each other and taught each other and commiserated when challenges arose and when a good outcome could not be attained, but they had gone into different disciplines. Clark practiced community general surgery, healing thousands of patients in a shoreline town. John had entered academic cardiac surgery.

Rarely did their professional spheres intersect.

Clark was calling about a patient, a healthy forty-five-year-old man. The last five years, his cardiologist had heard a murmur of mitral insufficiency. It hadn't bothered him at all, and no medications or restrictions of activity had been required. The patient continued an active lifestyle, even jogging five miles three times a week.

In the last few months, the patient couldn't run anymore. His wind just wasn't good enough. Lately, even walking to his office from the parking garage, he got short of breath. An echocardiogram had shown an increase in the degree of leakage of the mitral valve. Also, the left ventricle was starting to dilate—not a good sign. The cardiologist had recommended a valve repair operation.

"Would you be willing to do the operation?" asked Clark. Sure, John indicated, wondering why a general surgeon would be involved. "Of course I'll do it, Clark. How can I reach the patient?"

"You're talking to him," Clark said.

How many valves does the heart have?

There are four valves in your heart, two on the right side and two on the left side. (See the figures in the introduction.) The right side of the heart pumps blood to your lungs. The left side pumps blood to your body. There are two valves on the right side and two on the left side. The ones on the right side are the tricuspid and the pulmonic. These are of lesser importance, as the right side is the low-pressure side of the heart. Many people already know that the blood pressure in the arteries is about 120/80. The higher number is the *systolic* pressure, or the pressure during systole, the time when the heart muscle is contracting. The lower number is the *diastolic* pressure, or the pressure during diastole, the time when the heart muscle is resting. On the right side of the heart, the blood pressure is only about 25/10. You can see why the loads are less on the right side, and why valve surgery is rarely necessary on the right side.

You can review the normal appearance of the heart valves in the figures in the introduction.

On the left side, the important side, the two valves are called the *mitral* and the *aortic*. One easy way to understand these valves is to recognize that the mitral is the inflow valve into the main pumping chamber (the left ventricle) and that the aortic is the outflow valve from the main pumping chamber. Both are very, very important. Just picture any mechanical pump, like the water pump in your car. Imagine the excess load that valve dysfunction would place on any pump.

If the inflow valve, the mitral valve, is blocked, then blood cannot enter the left ventricle freely and easily. If the inflow valve is leaky, then blood will go *backward* through this valve when the heart contracts. You can easily picture that this cannot be good.

If the outflow valve, the aortic valve, is blocked, then blood cannot exit the heart freely and easily. It is almost as if your heart is being "strangled." If the outflow valve is leaky, then blood propelled forward by cardiac contraction runs *backward* into the heart again. This is also very bad. Your poor heart is burdened like the mythological character Sisyphus. (As we mentioned in the introduction, this is the unfortunate character from Greek mythology who was condemned to roll a heavy stone up a large hill, only to have it roll back as soon as he reached the top.) That is exactly the strain your heart suffers with a leaky valve; it has to pump the same blood over and over again out of your heart.

With these understandings, we have actually arrived at simple descriptions of the four conditions that can affect your heart valves and require surgery. These are shown in the following table.

Table 4.1. Conditions Affecting Heart Valves.

	Aortic	**Mitral**
Blocked	Aortic stenosis	Mitral stenosis
Leaky	Aortic regurgitation	Mitral regurgitation

The medical term for the condition wherein a valve is blocked is stenosis, from the Greek word for "narrow." The medical term for a condition wherein a valve is leaky is *regurgitation*, which means "backward flow of blood." The word *insufficiency* is sometimes substituted for *regurgitation*.

What is mitral stenosis?

Mitral stenosis is the narrowing of the inflow valve of the left ventricle. It is almost always caused by rheumatic fever that would have occurred decades earlier. Mitral stenosis puts a great strain on the lungs, as blood and pressure back up into the lungs as a consequence of the blockage at the level of the mitral valve. The left ventricle is protected and does not deteriorate over time, as it receives little load through the blocked mitral valve.

The following figure shows an example of mitral stenosis.

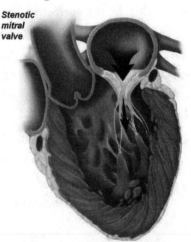

Stenotic mitral valve

Figure 4.1. Mitral stenosis. Note that only a small stream of blood (small arrow) is able to get through the narrowed orifice of the stenotic mitral valve.

What is mitral regurgitation?

Mitral regurgitation is the leaking (backward) of the mitral valve, the main inflow valve of the heart. The lungs are flooded. The left ventricle is strained and often damaged by having to pump an excess of blood because so much blood leaks backward.

The following figure shows an example of mitral regurgitation.

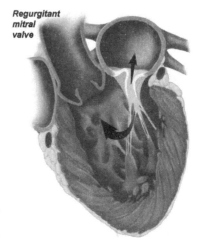

Regurgitant
mitral
valve

Figure 4.2. Mitral regurgitation. Note the abnormal stream of blood passing backwards through the mitral valve.

Case 2: Your Author, the "Stupidest" Person in the Room.

The author felt he was the "stupidest" person in the room. That was not a common feeling for him. But he was in a room with two dozen university physicists. His patient had invited him to a party at his house. The author couldn't help but ask for opinions, over drinks, from the assembled guests about nagging questions like the origins of the universe and how the pyramids were built.

Professor Erlich was eighty-two. "I still run two labs, one right here and one in Los Alamos," the professor had indicated to Dr. Elefteriades when he came for his pre-operative office visit. And he looked vigorous enough to justify the claim—tall, well built, moving like a much younger man. And, in terms of his mind, to say that it was "intact" despite his eighty-two years was an understatement. He had been considered for a Nobel Prize for his work. "I could tell you what I do," he told Dr. Elefteriades, "but you couldn't understand it." This was not arrogance, just a simple truth.

In the last few weeks, the professor had started getting a twinge of pain in his chest as he ran about the lab. Once, he had gotten lightheaded after working in the yard. On another occasion, he had awakened at night short of breath and had gone to the window for air. He called Dr. Cohen, who could tell from the professor's description that the narrowing of the aortic valve had finally started to impair Professor Erlich's heart.

Dr. Cohen saw the patient in his office. The murmur had gotten louder, even taking on a musical quality due to the excess velocity of blood flow through the narrowed valve. Since the opening was smaller, the blood needed to move faster. The echocardiogram confirmed that due to wear and tear—after all, his valve was eighty-two years old, like the rest of the professor—the aortic valve had become replete with calcium. The normally delicate, gossamer valve leaflets had, in essence, turned to bone. It could happen to anyone at that age. And, as the echo showed, the narrowing had attained a critical severity. Normally the size of a large garden hose, the aortic valve had been reduced to the dimensions of an eraser on the back of a lead pencil.

Surgery, Dr. Cohen had indicated to Professor Erlich, was the only option—a mechanical solution for an intrinsically mechanical problem. The renowned physicist understood, and thus began his relationship with the author.

What is aortic stenosis?

Aortic stenosis is the narrowing of the aortic valve, the main outflow valve of the heart. This places a great strain on the heart, "choking" it, in effect. This is a very damaging lesion (or abnormality).

The figures that follow show an example of aortic stenosis. The

Figures 4.3a and 4.3b. Aortic stenosis. Figure a shows the general appearance of aortic stenosis. Note that only a small stream of blood (small arrow) is able to pass through the narrowed aortic valve. This condition is so common and so significant that we show further details in part a of figure 4.3b. This figure shows how we approach the aortic valve by making a transverse incision in the aorta. Part b of figure 4.3b shows the typical appearance of calcific deposits on the valve leaflets, limiting their excursion. Part c of figure 4.3b shows, by way of contrast, a normal aortic valve seen through this same approach.

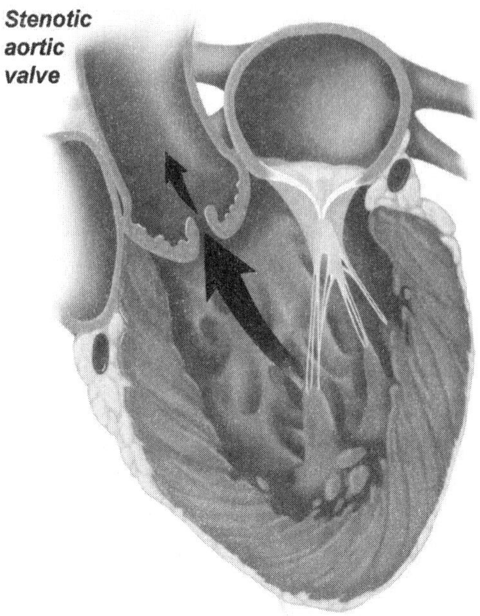

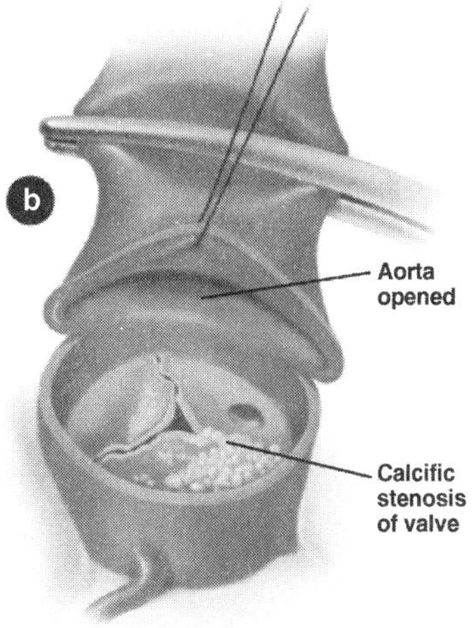

Stenotic aortic valve

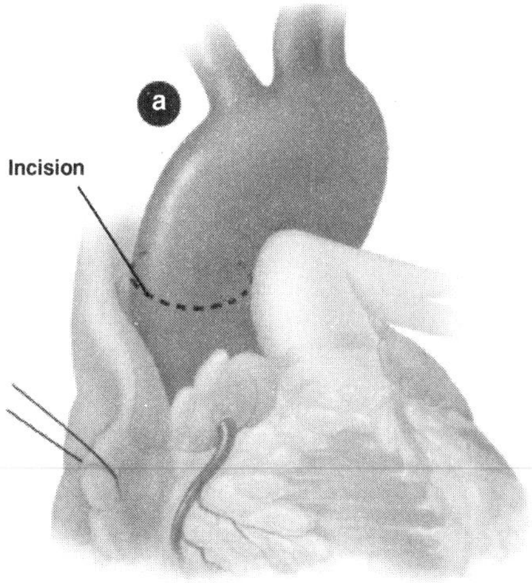

Incision

a

b

Aorta opened

Calcific stenosis of valve

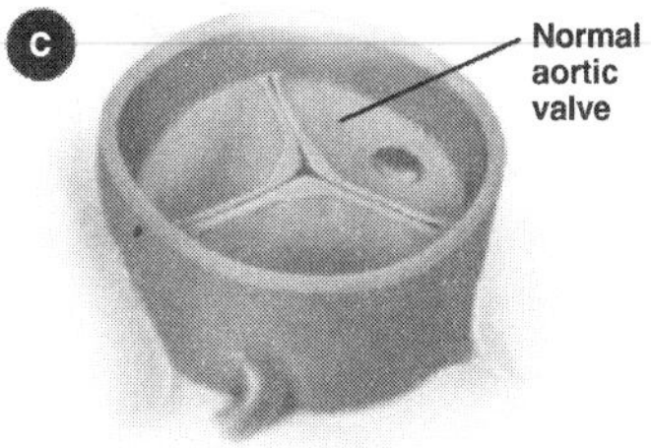

c

Normal aortic valve

buildup of calcium is very common in this condition. This is a vivid example of the "mechanical" nature of valve disease. No medication in the world can remove the bonelike calcium deposits that have developed on this valve.

What is aortic regurgitation?

Aortic regurgitation is the leaking of the aortic valve, the main outflow valve of the heart. This lesion places a great strain on the heart, forcing it to pump large volumes because so much blood leaks backward into the heart after being first ejected from the heart chambers.

The figure shows an example of blood leaking backward through a leaky aortic valve.

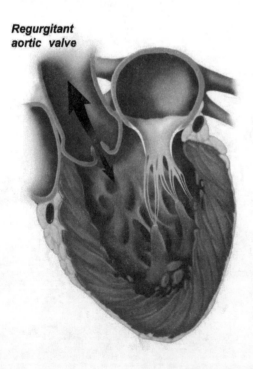

Regurgitant aortic valve

Figure 4.4. Aortic regurgitation. Note the abnormal stream of blood (small arrow) passing backward through the aortic valve.

What causes valve disease?

There are multiple causes of valve disease:

Birth defects. We may be born with disease of our valves. This can be part of a spectrum of congenital heart diseases that are outside the scope of this book.

Wear and tear. Valves can become diseased through the course of the normal wear and tear of life. Imagine that your heart beats, and each valve opens and closes 70 times a minute, 60 minutes per hour, 24 hours a day, 365 days a year, for the 75 years or more of your lifetime. This amounts to an astonishing 2.76 billion openings and closings per valve. No mechanical structure could tolerate such a load. Our hearts and valves are so exquisitely durable because the proteins that account for their structure are "turned over," or replaced, on a regular schedule throughout life. However, after years and years of service, anyone's valves can wear out. This is especially true for the aortic valve. This valve can become calcified and narrowed by the time even otherwise normal individuals reach their seventies or eighties. If an individual happens to be born with two instead of the normal three leaflets of the aortic valve, the valve is likely to wear out a decade or two earlier, that is, by the sixties or seventies.

Degeneration. In the case of the mitral valve, there is a condition that we call *degenerative valve disease* for want of a better term. Even in early or middle age, the delicate structures that make up the leaflets and chords of the mitral valve apparatus can become weakened or torn, leading to leaking of the mitral valve.

Infection. Valves can become infected. This happens when bacteria flood the bloodstream, as from a neglected boil or abscess. The teeth and oral cavity are frequent culprits in permitting dissemination of bacteria into the bloodstream. An infected valve will often perforate, leading to a backward leak of blood. The bacteria may form a clump, called a *vegetation*, on the edge of the valve leaflet. This vegetation may break off, or "embolize," damaging other organs downstream. Infection of a valve is called *endocarditis*. Often the term *bacterial endocarditis* is used, indicating the infectious origin of the problem. Endocarditis is a serious problem, requiring at a minimum weeks of continuous antibiotic therapy. Surgery is often required. In extreme cases, the infection may even destroy the very core of the heart, which may even become inoperable.

Rheumatic fever. The childhood infection rheumatic fever can cause valve disease decades later. The classic sequel of rheumatic fever is mitral stenosis.

Heart attack. A heart attack can result in leakage of the mitral valve, as the heart muscle itself is the motive force that closes the mitral valve apparatus.

Miscellaneous. A number of other conditions—including mitral valve prolapse (laxity of the valve structure), Marfan syndrome (an inherited condition), Ehler-Danlos syndrome (an inherited condition), and rheumatoid arthritis (a severe form of joint disease)—can at times cause heart valve disease. In very severe trauma, such as from a car accident, the heart valves may be ruptured or otherwise injured.

My best friend was just diagnosed with mitral valve prolapse. What does that mean?

Mitral valve prolapse (MVP) is a very common condition that in general is not dangerous. By some estimates, as many as ten percent of individuals may have it. It is more common in women than in men. It is a condition that is present at birth but may not come to light until the patient is in the teenage years or beyond. The abnormality relates to the mitral valve, which is abnormally large and may in time not close properly, thereby allowing leakage back from the left ventricle to the left atrium.

The characteristic physical finding when a doctor examines a patient with mitral valve prolapse is a midsystolic click, sometimes followed by a murmur. When there is a suspicion that a patient may have mitral valve prolapse, an echocardiogram, an ultrasound exam of the heart, is the diagnostic test of choice.

Most patients with mitral valve prolapse are asymptomatic, but some patients experience atypical chest pain or palpitations. The chest pain is not due to coronary artery narrowing, and the palpitations do not always correlate with abnormal heart rhythms.

In general, mitral valve prolapse does not lead to any major cardiac difficulties, but a fraction of patients born with this condition may develop mitral valve regurgitation (leakage). This may eventually, over decades, become sufficiently severe to warrant mitral valve surgery. This surgery can often be a reconstruction of the mitral valve, without requiring a replacement. On occasion, mitral valve replacement may be necessary. Although the need for surgery occurs in only a fraction of patients born with mitral valve prolapse, mitral valve prolapse has replaced rheumatic heart disease as the most common reason for mitral valve replacement.

There is some question surrounding whether a patient with a clear-cut click from mitral valve prolapse, but no murmur, requires prophylactic antibiotics before a dental procedure or other invasive intervention. We lean toward prescribing two grams of amoxicillin or other appropriate antibiotic before such a procedure. There is no question, however, whether antibiotics should be prescribed if the patient has a murmur in addition to a click. In all such instances, a prophylactic antibiotic is required. Patients who have mitral valve prolapse with a murmur are at risk of developing a heart valve infection following any type of dental procedure, colonoscopy, or other medical intervention that could trigger bacteria being released into the bloodstream.

I've been told that I was born with two leaflets in my aortic valve. What does that mean?

Most people have three leaflets in the aortic valve; this normal anatomy is therefore called a *tricuspid* valve. In some cases, the valve has only two leaflets; this makes it a *bicuspid* valve. This is actually one of the most common congenital heart irregularities, affecting fully one or two out of every hundred newborn children. The anomaly continues, of course, throughout life.

The diagnosis is usually made by an echocardiogram.

As mentioned above, it is a matter of amazement to ponder just how many times our heart valves open and close during a lifetime. It is truly astounding that any structure of any kind can sustain the intensity of use inherent in the billions of opening and closing excursions estimated previously.

In fact, in any of us, the aortic valve may "wear out" by the time we are seventy or eighty years of age. In those of us with bicuspid valves, wear and tear on the abnormal valve can cause it to deteriorate two decades earlier, by the time we are fifty or sixty years old. The valve may become regurgitant or stenotic—that is, leaky or blocked. In some people, the valve may become abnormal even in young adulthood or childhood.

We now know that some other abnormalities are often associated with bicuspid aortic valve. Patients with these abnormalities may also be affected by what we call coarctation of the aorta. In this condition, a membrane narrows the aorta in the part that descends toward the abdomen at the back of the chest. This membrane can produce a partial blockage that can affect flow of blood and blood pressure. Also, patients with bicuspid aortic valve may be vulnerable to what is called *aortic dissection*, a serious internal splitting of the aortic wall itself. (This is discussed more fully below.)

We now know that patients with bicuspid aortic valve may

suffer aortic dissection even before they become symptomatic with aortic regurgitation or aortic stenosis. Development of an enlarged aorta, or an *aortic aneurysm* (see below), often precedes aortic dissection.

You can tell from this discussion that if you are known to have a bicuspid aortic valve, you must be followed closely by your doctors. You must report any onset of symptoms, especially shortness of breath or chest pain, to your doctors promptly. With proper follow-up, you can be kept safe and sound with your doctors' help.

How is my valve disease related to my heart failure?

Valvular heart disease is one of the most common causes of heart failure. By the mechanisms indicated above—stenosis or regurgitation of the mitral or aortic valves—blood under pressure builds up in the lungs, leading to difficulty breathing. The heart enlarges, getting progressively weaker and weaker. The weak heart leads to fluid buildup throughout the body, most easily seen in the ankles. These events constitute the explicit manifestations of congestive heart failure.

I have aortic stenosis. My doctor keeps asking me if I'm getting dizzy or light-headed. What does dizziness have to do with my aortic valve?

When aortic stenosis is severe, it can limit the amount of blood flow that the heart can pump. If you suddenly change position or abruptly exert yourself, the instantaneous demand for blood flow may exceed what the heart can actually deliver through your narrowed aortic valve. The net result is dizziness or even loss of consciousness because blood flow to the brain is inadequate. This is a very serious symptom of aortic stenosis. This requires surgical replacement of your aortic valve.

HYPERTENSION, HIGH CHOLESTEROL, AND ARTERIOSCLEROSIS

High blood pressure (or hypertension) and a high cholesterol level have long been known to contribute to the development of hardening of the arteries, or arteriosclerosis. In this process, fatty deposits may develop in *any* of the arteries of the body. Virtually any blood vessels can be involved. Those of the heart, brain, and kidney are most important. Leg arteries are often involved, leading to claudication, or pain with walking. The intestinal arteries are less commonly involved, leading to intestinal angina or death of parts of the intestines. While these disturbances—hypertension, high cholesterol, and general arteriosclerosis—are not specifically cardiac diseases, they have a strong impact on the heart.

Case 1. Maria from Italy.

Maria had come from Italy at eighteen years of age. She had married a fellow immigrant shortly thereafter, and together they had raised four children, all of whom went on to distinguish themselves academically and professionally. She was seventy-eight years old.

She had been noted to have high blood pressure for many years, but she, as well as some of her physicians, had dismissed this as a "white coat syndrome." That is to say, some patients become anxious when their blood pressure is taken, which artificially elevates the readings. This was thought to be the case for Maria. Indeed, when her husband took the readings with a home blood pressure device, they were lower. In fact, Maria took her antihypertensive pills only irregularly for many years, and then stopped complying entirely. She saw her doctor only erratically and did not fully confide her medical noncompliance.

She found herself now in the neurologic intensive care unit. She had lost consciousness at home while cooking a Sunday dinner for her children and grandchil-dren. She had regained consciousness after arrival in the ICU, but her speech was slurred, she had trouble finding words, and she was weak on one side of her body. The neurologist suspected a stroke. The CT (computed tomography) scan confirmed the suspicion, showing a site of bleeding into the substance of the brain.

Her blood pressure on admission to the emergency room had been 210/150. The years of hypertension had finally taken their toll; one of the blood vessels in her brain had essentially "burst" from the excess tension within. Care at this point was merely supportive. It remained to be seen what extent of recovery would be realized.

What is blood pressure?

Blood pressure refers to the pressure within the major blood vessels of the body. It is measured by a device called a *sphygmomanometer*, or blood pressure cuff. The accompanying figure illustrates how a blood pressure cuff works.

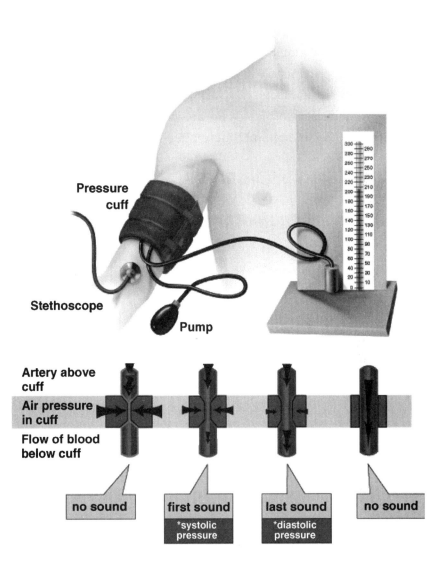

Figure 5.1. Blood pressure cuff.

Blood pressure is the end result of a complex set of normal events in the body. The left ventricle pumps blood from the heart into the aorta. The column of blood enters the aorta with a considerable amount of force. In the late eighteenth century, a clergyman named Stephen Hales inserted a cannula into an artery and noted that the arterial column rose approximately eight feet. The level of blood pressure is determined by several factors: (1) the pumping action of the heart, (2) the peripheral resistance, and (3) the amount of blood in the arteries.

Through the interaction of these three factors, blood pressure is determined. If the heart is pumping vigorously, as during exercise, the resistance in the vessels decreases so that the blood pressure stays within a normal range.

What is hypertension?
What do *systolic* and *diastolic* mean?

The pressure within the large blood vessels defines whether or not an individual has a normal or an elevated blood pressure. If the blood pressure exceeds 140/90 millimeters of mercury (abbreviated mmHg), this is defined as hypertension. Ideally, however, the blood pressure should be lower—in the 120 to 130/70 to 75 mmHg range. The first number of the blood pressure is the *systolic* blood pressure and the second number is the *diastolic* blood pressure. *Systolic* refers to the pressure when the heart muscle is contracting, and *diastolic* refers to the pressure when the heart muscle is relaxed (see the section titled "How many valves does the heart have?" in chapter 4). The use of millimeters of mercury as a measure of blood pressure has become traditional; this measure refers to the height to which a column of mercury (a heavy liquid metal) would be lifted if exposed to the pressure of the blood.

One or the other of these numbers may be elevated, and if it is, the patient has hypertension or high blood pressure. With aging, it is quite normal for the systolic blood pressure to become elevated. Once it was believed that this was a normal concomitant of aging. More recent studies, however, point to this form of elevated blood pressure as being less than desirable and not necessarily normal. Another type of blood pressure abnormality is called labile hypertension. This condition is characterized by wide swings in blood pressure over short periods of time. The natural history of patients with labile hypertension often leads to more fixed hypertension as they get older.

How can hypertension cause heart disease?

Hypertension puts a strain on the blood vessels, accelerating the arteriosclerotic process. Also, hypertension places an excess load on the main pumping chamber of the heart. The heart wall becomes thick and muscle-bound, a condition known as hypertrophy. This condition is quite harmful. Such a heart requires excess blood flow. Moreover, such a heart becomes abnormally stiff.

What causes hypertension?

In the majority of cases, the cause of hypertension is not known. In a minority of patients who develop hypertension, there may be a hormonal reason, such as an overactive adrenal gland causing hyperaldosteronism or an adrenal tumor called a pheochromocytoma. Similarly, abnormalities of the pituitary or adrenal glands may lead to Cushing's syndrome, a condition of excess steroid hormones accompanied by hypertension. A congenital abnormality of the aorta, called a *coarctation*, is responsible for a small number of cases of hypertension. But the vast majority of cases of hypertension occur with no currently known cause. Genetics is a factor, lifestyle is a factor, and diet is a factor, but often there are no known contributing causes. Fortunately, the vast majority of cases can be treated with medications, thereby preventing the damage that uncontrolled hypertension may cause—arteriosclerosis, stroke, heart attack, and kidney failure, among other consequences.

Is hypertension hereditary?

There is not a one-to-one relationship between heredity and hypertension, but there is a tendency for hypertension to run in families. There may be individuals who develop hypertension in spite of no family history and others who do not develop hypertension in spite of a strong family history.

What is a coarctation of the aorta?

A coarctation, or narrowing, of the aorta is a congenital abnormality of the aorta, the major blood vessel that carries blood from the heart to the rest of the body. The area of narrowing is usually located at the site where the aorta starts its downward course in the upper back or thoracic area. The narrowing is usually not a complete one, but it may be of such a severity that blood vessels (collaterals) grow around it, so that the lower portion of the body can receive an adequate blood supply. These collateral vessels, as they enlarge, will at times erode into the posterior rib cage and cause "notching," which will be visible on a chest X-ray. The therapy for a patient who has a coarctation is usually surgical, but of late, some coarctations can be approached by balloon angioplasty. Correction by either means should be performed whenever the abnormality is diagnosed, since the hypertension caused by the narrowing is often deleterious to vessels supplying the brain. The correction of coarctation usually cures the hypertension, although some patients do not completely lose their hypertension and require continuing antihypertensive medications.

Case 2. High Blood Pressure and Low Kidney Function.

Arnold Kramer was incredulous. "Dialysis" the doctor had said, or "a kidney transplant." Arnold and his wife could not believe their ears.

Sure, he had had high blood pressure since he was forty. He was now sixty-five, and proud that he had never spent a day in a hospital. Yes, he remembered that the doctor had told him that his "kidney chemicals" were abnormal on his yearly blood tests. He vaguely remembered the doctor explaining that high blood pressure, over long periods of time, was harmful to the kidneys. The doctor reiterated this at today's visit.

Now, the doctor had said, his "creatinine" was 5. Normal was 1. Last year, Arnold's level had been 2.5. Creatinine is a waste product normally cleared by the kidneys. Now, the kidneys were failing severely. This explained the lethargy that had prompted Arnold's current visit to his doctor. His nausea and lack of appetite were consequences as well. The doctor was surprised that Arnold had not been feeling even worse.

Mrs. Kramer was insistent that the doctor do something to correct the situation. Surely, she thought, the blood pressure could be controlled and the kidney function would improve. Not so, the doctor explained. The damage was cumulative, progressing year after year. At this point, the damage to the kidneys was irreversible. Either dialysis, with the machine providing the blood cleansing normally performed by the kidneys, or kidney transplantation were required.

The doctor wanted to admit Arnold, but, headstrong as Arnold was, he preferred to consider his options from home. He promised to return a few days later for another blood test to make sure that no life-threatening chemical abnormalities had developed.

What organs can be damaged by hypertension?

Hypertension damages *all* the blood vessels in the body. And *all* of our internal organs depend on blood vessels for the delivery of oxygen and nutrients. But it is the brain, the kidneys, and the heart that are most vulnerable. The brain may suffer strokes, the kidneys may suffer failure, and the heart may suffer angina or heart attack.

Case 3. The Devastation of Juvenile Diabetes.

I thought the wrong patient had walked into my office for the consultation. The appearance of the patient seemed incongruous with the catheterization films I had just reviewed.

The films showed extremely advanced coronary artery disease. The LAD, the most important branch artery of the heart, supplying the whole front of the heart muscle, was 99 percent blocked near its origin. The circumflex coronary artery, supplying the left side of the heart, was also 99 percent blocked. The lesions were so tight that it appeared that the red blood cells would have to line up one by one, stand in line single file, and turn side-ways to make their way through the blockage in order to reach the heart muscle. (We are speaking figuratively here, of course, but not exaggerating by much.) And the only other main coronary artery, the right coronary artery, which supplies the back of the heart, was already "down," having closed who knows how long ago. In addition, there was what we call diffuse coronary artery disease. That is, instead of discrete, localized blockages at the top of the arteries, the whole length of each vessel was diseased, with a ratty, irregular appearance signifying intense involvement of the entire vessel—top to bottom—by arteriosclerosis. The only good finding on the catheterization films was that the heart muscle itself was remarkably strong; it showed a totally normal squeezing pattern when it filled with dye from the catheter. Fortunately, the blocked arteries had not yet taken a toll on the heart muscle itself.

From the catheterization, I anticipated an extremely elderly woman. It normally takes decades to produce the severe, extensive pattern of blockages that I saw on the angiogram. And women do not even start the process until after menopause.

But the woman I saw walk in was trim, tanned, muscular, well dressed, well appointed, and young. She looked the picture of health. I could tell from her trim, lithe body that she was a runner. Was she the daughter? No—no one else walked into the room, and this young woman closed the door behind her.

It turned out that the ninety-year-old–appearing coronary arteries I had seen were hers. I checked the birth date in my file, finding that she was only thirty-seven years old.

How could this be? What explained this incongruity?

Well, in all his practice, the author had seen only a handful of cases in which a premenopausal woman had developed coronary artery disease severe enough to require a bypass procedure. Those women invariably had one of two illnesses: either juvenile onset diabetes (the extremely severe type of diabetes that begins in childhood) or familial hyperlipidemia (an inherited, severe form of high blood fats). Nancy, it turned, had both. She had developed diabetes when she was seven years old; she could not remember life without insulin injections. And, to make matters worse, her cholesterol was 375 and her triglycerides were 400. Her blood was literally laden with fats. Her father and her brother had it as well. Between the high fats and the effects of the diabetes, her coronary arteries did not have a chance. This is how she came to have ninety-year-old arteries in a thirty-seven-year-old body.

She had been running two to three miles a day until this month. She didn't have chest pain, not even at the peak of exertion, the diabetes having numbed the nerves that would normally have alerted her to heart disease years ago. All she felt was a decrease in her exercise tolerance. She was excessively concerned about her appearance. This is why she had sought medical attention. She was afraid that if she wasn't able to run more than she could currently manage, she would gain weight.

She saw her general doctor, who astutely suspected heart disease, despite the outward appearances. She was referred to a cardiologist. Her exercise test (running on a treadmill) showed severe, threatening EKG changes, and she underwent the catheterization that demonstrated the severe, diffuse three-vessel coronary artery disease.

And now she was in the office to discuss and plan a coronary bypass operation—at the young age of thirty-seven.

What is cholesterol?

Despite its bad reputation, cholesterol is an essential substance for human life. This fatty substance is manufactured in the liver and serves several vital functions in the body's chemistry. Without cholesterol, the body could not produce the steroid and sex hormones that regulate body functions or the bile that is essential for digesting our foods.

How do high cholesterol levels lead to heart disease?

High cholesterol levels promote arteriosclerosis. When arteriosclerosis affects the coronary arteries—those that provide blood supply to the heart muscle itself—angina or heart attack may be the end result.

I maintain a healthy diet, but my doctors say that my cholesterol level is too high. How can this be?

The level of cholesterol that an individual manifests is determined by a number of factors. Genetics is one of those factors. There are individuals who inherit a gene that may lead to a higher than normal cholesterol. Their livers manufacture cholesterol from surplus biochemical products. Similarly, other individuals inherit a gene that does not permit the body to rid itself of cholesterol. Therefore, some individuals, those with these hereditary patterns, may have an elevated cholesterol level even if their diet is virtually fat- and cholesterol-free.

Still other individuals may have elevated cholesterol because of a diet that is high in saturated fats and cholesterol. In a society that emphasizes fast foods, this may be especially true. Good eating habits should be learned early in life and carried forward into adulthood.

What is meant by "good" and "bad" cholesterol?

The total cholesterol value is made up of several components. The two most important components are low-density lipoprotein (LDL) and high-density lipoprotein (HDL).

The LDL cholesterol is referred to as the "bad" cholesterol, and the HDL cholesterol is referred to as the "good" cholesterol. This is because LDL cholesterol is associated with the development of coronary artery disease. It has been known for many years that high LDL cholesterol is correlated with heart attacks. HDL cholesterol, on the other hand, is protective. It functions to help transport bad cholesterol out of the body. Ordinarily, LDL cholesterol makes up a significant portion of total cholesterol. Therefore, individuals with high total cholesterol usually have high LDL cholesterol. HDL cholesterol makes up a smaller fraction of total cholesterol, usually just 20 to 25 percent. However, in certain individuals, particularly premenopausal women, HDL cholesterol may be quite a bit more abundant. In these instances, a high level of total cholesterol is of lesser prognostic significance.

My doctor says I have high triglycerides. What does this mean?

A separate lipid (or fatty) component of the blood is a substance called triglycerides. Its role in the development of coronary atherosclerosis (hardening of the arteries of the heart) is of lesser importance. There is a weak association between high triglycerides and coronary disease. However, individuals with high levels of triglycerides usually have concomitant elevations of cholesterol. Therefore, high triglycerides are often a marker for predisposition to coronary disease. Individuals with very high levels of triglycerides are susceptible to developing pancreatitis, at times a life-threatening problem. Also, patients with diabetes often have high levels of triglycerides. Weight gain and alcohol consumption tend to raise triglycerides, whereas exercise, weight loss, and abstinence from alcohol tend to lower triglycerides. The goal is to keep your triglycerides level below two hundred.

What is the relationship between high cholesterol and coronary artery disease?

In 1948 the government started a study called the Framingham Heart Study, named for the town of Framingham, Massachusetts. All fifty thousand inhabitants of Framingham were examined and had extensive blood work done. They were then followed up and examined annually. The town of Framingham was chosen because it had a relatively stable population and was near the medical center that undertook the study. One of the early and abiding results to come from the Framingham Study indicated that there was a predictable increase in the development of heart attacks over the years in proportion to how much the cholesterol levels were above 200 milligrams per decileter. Although most of the adult population is now aware of the link between cholesterol and heart disease, it was not known before the Framingham Study made its first report. Although the mechanism by which high cholesterol leads to heart attacks is a complex one, it is certainly mediated through cholesterol's forming a major component of plaques or narrowing in the coronary arteries.

How can I lower my cholesterol?

Cholesterol levels are in large part genetically determined. Although we cannot choose our parents, there are ways in which cholesterol levels can be lowered. Diet—the type of food one eats—is important. Foods such as meat—especially fatty meats, sweetbreads, and many forms of fast food such as hamburgers, fried foods, or pizza—contribute to raising cholesterol levels. Foods such as fish, lean chicken, salads, and liquid rather than solid fats and oils tend to lower cholesterol. Weight loss to an optimal range for one's size will generally lower cholesterol. Regular exercise, at least three times a week, will also lower cholesterol. Moreover, there have been a number of medications developed over the years that have a predictable action on lowering cholesterol.

Are there other benefits to lowering my cholesterol?

There is actually very recent emerging, but compelling, evidence that lowering cholesterol may actually decrease the likelihood of developing Alzheimer's disease late in life. The evidence shows that individuals genetically prone to Alzheimer's disease do much better if their cholesterol is kept in line by diet, exercise, or medications.

I am a forty-year-old woman. My total cholesterol is 280 milligrams per deciliter, but my "good" cholesterol (HDL) is 80 milligrams per deciliter. Do I have to worry?

Many premenopausal women are blessed with a high level of HDL cholesterol, the good cholesterol. In a number of ways this cholesterol is protective and helps prevent development of plaque in the coronary arteries. As a simple way of assessing whether an individual is at increased risk, the ratio of total cholesterol divided by HDL cholesterol is calculated. A ratio of less than 4:1 is desirable. In the case of a patient with a total cholesterol of 280 milligrams per deciliter and an HDL cholesterol of 80 milligrams per deciliter, the ratio would be 3:5. Thus, your cholesterol profile is satisfactory. As menopause occurs, it is usual for HDL cholesterol levels to fall. If this does occur, it would be prudent to lower your total cholesterol through medication, in addition to diet and exercise.

Can you explain low lipid levels and other goals to me?

In terms of other goals, we now recommend that the LDL level be maintained below one hundred milligrams per deciliter. This is a much stricter criterion than those recommended as recently as a decade ago. We are recommending stringent cholesterol control because we have recognized more and more the importance of cholesterol as a risk factor for development of coronary artery disease. For certain patients, like those who have suffered a heart attack, it may even be best to aim for a level as low as 75 for your LDL cholesterol.

In terms of HDL cholesterol, your level should ideally be above 40 milligrams per deciliter in order for this good cholesterol to protect you from fatty buildup in your arteries.

These numbers, 130 for LDL and 40 for HDL, mean that your total cholesterol should be 170 or less.

One important goal is to attain an HDL cholesterol level one-quarter or more of the total cholesterol level. This recommendation is a reflection of the fact that HDL is good cholesterol.

These goals are illustrated in the accompanying table. Cholesterol is measured in milligrams per deciliter, abbreviated mg/dl.

Upon reaching adulthood, individuals should have their cholesterol level checked once every few years.

Table 5.1. Cholesterol Levels.

Parameter	Goals	
	Adequate	Ideal
Total cholesterol	< 200 mg/dl	< 150 mg/dl
HDL (good cholesterol)	> 40 mg/dl	> 45 mg/dl
LDL (bad cholesterol)	< 130 mg/dl	< 100 mg/dl
Triglycerides	< 200 mg/dl	< 150 mg/dl

The accompanying figure illustrates the goals to be attained in lipid control.

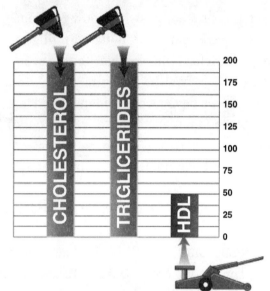

Figure 5.2. Beating down the "bad" cholesterol and triglycerides, and pumping up the "good" HDL.

I have heard that cholesterol and triglycerides are only part of the lipid story, that there are other important blood factors being discovered. Can you tell me about these?

You are indeed correct. Medical science is discovering multiple additional circulating blood chemicals that can help to predict which patients are especially likely to develop coronary artery disease or to suffer heart attacks. Many doctors are not yet monitoring these other blood factors routinely. Sometimes, your health plan may not cover these tests, whose importance is only now emerging into medical consciousness.

In particular, there are seven subtypes of bad LDL cholesterol. Two of them are especially bad. One of these subtypes, called *small, dense lipoprotein*, increases your risk of events by 300 percent.

Another subtype of LDL, lipoprotein (a), or Lp(a), is also highly predictive of adverse cardiac events.

The test for C-reactive protein can, in some cases, predict coronary artery disease years in advance.

Some of these other factors are itemized in the accompanying table. Your doctor may check some of these factors in your case. You may also ask your doctor about some of these tests, if you are interested in predicting your risk extremely accurately. These tests permit a more thorough analysis of your risk of cardiac events than the simple HDL, LDL, and triglyceride tests. Drs. Thomas Yannios and Robert Superko have written extensively about these alternate risk factors.

Table 5.2. Alternate Risk Factors.

	Description	**Impact**	**Goal levels**
Lipoprotein (a)	Also called Lp(a) or "lipoprotein little a"	Increases risk 70 percent	< 20 mg/dl
Small, dense lipoprotein	Likely to burrow into artery	Increases risk 300 percent	< 15.6 percent
Apoprotein B	Like a cap on lipo particles		< 107 mg/dl
Fibrinogen	Makes blood thick, clot-like	Increases risk 200 percent	< 324 mg/dl
C-reactive protein	Marker of inflamation	Increases risk 400 percent	< 0.07 mg/dl
Homocysteine	Promotes clotting	Increases risk 400 percent	< 11.6 micromol/ liter

What is that new test I keep hearing about that is better than a cholesterol check?

You have probably heard about the C-reactive protein test, one of the blood studies mentioned in the table above. This factor in the blood is a marker of inflammation in the body. Remember that inflammation is a medical term for irritation. Infection can be one cause of inflammation. Inflammation can have many other causes besides infection. In many cases, the body simply becomes irritated with its own tissues. In the case of heart disease, we do not know conclusively whether the inflammation detected by the C-reactive protein is due to internal irritation or to an occult infection, bacterial or viral, hiding somewhere in the body.

In any case, the C-reactive protein test is an inexpensive, simple, readily available blood investigation that can accurately predict your risk of coronary artery disease. You are entirely correct that heart specialists are focusing more and more on this blood test, in addition to cholesterol and lipid levels. Monitoring the C-reactive protein for clinical purposes is relatively recent, but the enthusiasm is very high. If the C-reactive protein level is low, the risk of heart attack is low. If the C-reactive protein level is high, the risk of heart attack is high.

We believe that C-reactive protein levels are so strongly predictive because they provide an index of the degree of ambient inflammation in our bodies. Such inflammation probably plays an important role in allowing a clot to form at the site of an arteriosclerotic plaque in a coronary artery, which produces a heart attack.

The accompanying figure (fig. 5.3) shows how your doctor can use both the cholesterol and C-reactive protein levels to accurately predict your risk of heart attack. Note that while your heart attack risk rises with increases in either LDL cholesterol or CRP, the rise with CRP is even more pronounced.

hs-CRP is a stronger predictor of heart attack and stroke than LDL cholesterol

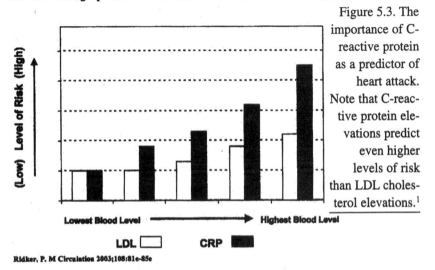

Figure 5.3. The importance of C-reactive protein as a predictor of heart attack. Note that C-reactive protein elevations predict even higher levels of risk than LDL cholesterol elevations.[1]

Ridker, P. M Circulation 2003;108:81e-85e

To summarize, C-reactive protein will not replace cholesterol measurement, but at this time it appears to be an extremely important part of our armamentarium for predicting your cardiac risk. Your authors expect that C-reactive protein will soon become a household word.

Case 4. Arteriosclerosis Everywhere.

Mr. Amarante, seventy-five years old, represented the ravages of arteriosclerosis at full tilt. Our team was called to see him in the coronary care unit, where he was on IV nitroglycerine to control his chest pain.

He had worked as a tool maker in New London, a nearby town known for its building of submarines and other high-tech weapons of war and defense. He had been at the same ship-building employer for thirty-five years. He had retired at age sixty-five. He had smoked since he was thirteen. His mother had had a bypass at seventy-three years of age. His brother had already had two bypass operations, the first one fifteen years ago, and the second the previous year.

Mr. Amarante had enjoyed the first five years of his retirement. The next five were not as good. He had suffered from angina during that time. He had required one angioplasty to clear a blocked artery in his heart. He was on a host of medications to keep the angioplasty open and to keep his heart rate and blood pressure controlled.

We were called to see him for an urgent coronary artery bypass operation. He had been admitted with chest pain. The chest pain had been controlled by nitroglycerine. He had had a catheterization, showing disease of all three of his coronary arteries. There was a moderate amount of muscle damage, visible in the decreased strength of contraction of his heart muscle.

The young resident sur-

geon who first saw him returned to the author with a number of concerns, all of them well placed. Basically, they all had to do with evidence of arteriosclerosis at other sites in addition to the heart.

It turns out that in addition to the chest pains, the patient had suffered several TIAs, or transient ischemic attacks. This is a technical term referring to ministrokes, or strokes of the brain that resolve spontaneously without permanent sequellae. The first had occurred three years ago. According to his wife, Mary, Mr. Amarante had slumped down to the kitchen floor when he attempted to rise from the dinner table. His left leg went numb and weak. He could not move his left arm. His speech was slurred, and the right corner of his mouth drooped. He was confused and not in control of himself. Mary had summoned the ambulance, and by the time he arrived at the emergency room, Mr.

Amarante was already improving. By the time the neurologist arrived, there were no abnormal findings. A CT scan of the brain was, thank goodness, normal—no brain damage was evident. An echo exam of the brain arteries showed an 80 percent blockage of the right carotid artery, the one leading to the right side of the brain, which controls motion on the left side of the body. The patient was started on aspirin to thin the blood so it could flow more easily through the narrowed carotid artery. Surgery for the carotid artery had been mentioned, but Mr. Amarante was not enthusiastic. An earlier episode had occurred during the previous year's Thanksgiving holiday, and, the patient explained, he had a brief attack just last week. Each time, the effects were similar—weakness of the left arm and leg being the most prominent symptoms. Fortunately, the episodes after the initial one had lasted only minutes. The family recognized the symptoms, and all they did was call the doctor. Mr. Amarante didn't even come to the hospital for the brief TIAs. To the family, the episodes were not of great concern, but to our resident they were. He recognized these episodes as reflecting transient inadequacy of blood flow to the brain—a serious state of affairs, especially in a patient being evaluated for heart surgery. The surgery would certainly put a strain on the brain. A stroke could result.

The resident also learned that for the last year Mr. Amarante had suffered pain in his right calf when he walked more than two blocks. The calf cramped up and Mr. A. had to rest before continuing. The resident recognized this as intermittent claudication, the technical term indicating that blood flow to the leg was inadequate under load. On examining Mr. A., the resident easily discerned why: the femoral (or groin) pulse was weak on that side. And none of the normal pulses below that level—behind the knee, behind the ankle, or on the top of the foot—were even remotely discernible. Clearly, the blood vessels to the right lower extremity were occluded (totally blocked).

The other factor with which the resident surgeon was not pleased was the serum creatinine. This blood test measures the level of a chemical normally cleared by the kidneys. Normal is up to 1.5. Mr. A.'s creatinine was 2.5. That may not sound too bad, but actually that level indicates that arteriosclerotic deposits in the small arteries of the kidneys had robbed Mr. A. of 85 percent of the kidney function with which he had been born.

So, the resident reported, he had found evidence that arteriosclerosis had ravaged the blood vessels in multiple sites in Mr. A.'s body: not only the heart, but also the brain, the legs, and the kidneys. Unfortunately, this pattern of general involvement by the arteriosclerotic process was disturbingly common. None of this boded well for the patient's candidacy for cardiac surgery. And the resident recognized from his considerable experience that this was likely just the tip of the iceberg, with many more arterial deposits in other arteries yet to be detected.

What is arteriosclerosis?

Arteriosclerosis is the hardening of the arteries. In the case of the heart, arteriosclerosis causes blockages in the coronary arteries. It is the coronary arteries that are responsible for supplying blood flow to the heart muscle itself.

Arteriosclerosis is manifest as lipid deposition in the affected arteries. In the operating room, we can often see yellowish discoloration of involved arterial segments. In more severe zones, the artery wall actually becomes filled with the mineral calcium, which gives it a bone-hard consistency. Arteries should normally be softer than the pulp of your fingertip. When medical students touch and feel severely diseased coronary arteries in the operating room, they remark that the vessels are so rigid they feel more like some mechanical pipe rather than an internal part of a human being.

What causes arteriosclerosis?

Despite decades of intensive investigation, we still do not completely understand what causes arteriosclerosis. We know that excess fats in the bloodstream get deposited in the wall of arteries. We know that eating fatty foods and having high cholesterol levels contribute to the accumulation of these fatty deposits.

We also know that these fatty deposits are more likely to occur if the inner lining of the vessel—the endothelium (also called intima)—is injured. In effect, the inner lining is the guardian that prevents access of the lipids to the vessel wall. When this guardian is incapacitated, the vessel wall becomes vulnerable. We know that high blood pressure, stress, and cigarette smoking damage the endothelial guardian membrane. See the accompanying figure, which illustrates how the process of arteriosclerosis begins, from endothelial injury, and then progresses with lipid deposition.

We also know that genetics contributes to development of arteriosclerosis. A positive family history certainly renders one more susceptible. Yet this is not an exact, one-to-one relationship.

We do know that exercise is beneficial in preventing arteriosclerosis even in families that are susceptible to it.

In some sense, however, although we know so very much about

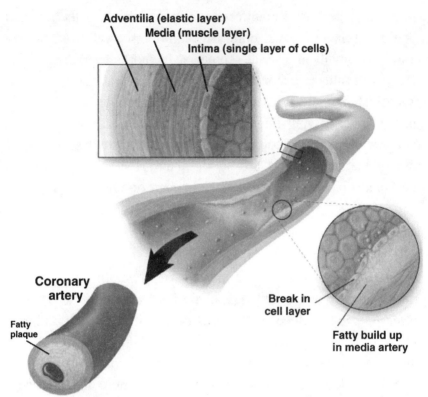

Figure 5.4. The process of arteriosclerosis, beginning with endothelial injury. The insert shows the break in the endothelium (intima) that permits the entry of fatty deposits into the deeper layers of the aortic wall.

the process of development of arteriosclerosis, the fundamental cause still eludes medical science. We do not know the fundamental trigger for all the causative associations mentioned above. Some medical professionals have even suggested that a chronic, smoldering bacterial infection of the arteries may be the fundamental cause. In that case, antibiotics might become a new treatment. After all, for decades medical science treated ulcers as acid phenomena, whereas we now know that a bacterium, Helicobacter pylori, is responsible; we now eradicate this disease by giving antibiotics.

The mystery of the ubiquitous and destructive process of arteriosclerosis still eludes complete clarification.

I've heard that arteriosclerosis may be caused by infection; what's the story on this?

There is preliminary yet mounting evidence to support this point of view. Specifically, patients with arteriosclerosis, especially coronary artery disease, have high levels of infectious indicators in the bloodstream. Also, in specimens of plaques taken from coronary arteries at the time of coronary artery surgery, it is quite common to find traces of bacteria and other germs. Furthermore, there has been some semblance of improvement in coronary artery patients treated with antibiotics in addition to their standard medications. However, this viewpoint still remains that of a minority of specialists, although support is building. The controversial but brilliant evolutionary microbiologist Dr. Paul Ewald of Amherst University tries to put himself into the "minds" of the microorganisms to understand how they could cause arteriosclerosis.[2] If the germ was really smart, Dr. Ewald maintains, it would not cause an illness immediately fatal to the host; to do so would result in eradication of the germ species. Rather, a smart germ would cause a long-standing, smoldering, low-grade infection that would not kill the host for a very long time. Thus, the germ can multiply its species with abundant time to be disseminated from one individual host to others. Arteriosclerosis, a long-smoldering disease, would certainly provide such a long window of opportunity to infectious organisms.

We, the authors, believe that within ten years, there may be general support for an infectious cause of arteriosclerosis, with new possibilities opened up for treatment and prevention.

I read that high iron levels are responsible for arteriosclerosis, and that women are protected by their regular monthly blood loss; what's the story on this?

It is a well-known fact that women are relatively protected from arteriosclerosis and coronary artery disease during their reproductive years. It is very, very rare for a premenopausal woman to need a coronary artery bypass operation. The only young female patients who need bypass surgery almost invariably have what we call juvenile onset diabetes—that is, Type I diabetes originating in childhood.

Despite intensive research, the reason women are protected has never been conclusively demonstrated. Some authorities have felt that the female hormones are somehow protective. Recently, some evidence has appeared indicating that iron may be one culprit in bringing on coronary artery disease. Because women lose iron monthly with their periods, they are protected from this possible damaging role of iron.

Suffice it to say, women are protected early on from coronary artery disease, and we do not know exactly why.

On the other hand, it is very important to be aware that, after menopause, women catch up very quickly with men in their propensity for coronary artery disease. Chest pain or other cardiac-type symptoms need to be examined and pursued aggressively regardless of the patient's gender. Traditionally, over the decades, heart disease has escaped detection in women simply because of their gender and the mistaken impression that women are less prone to cardiac disease.

My doctor mentioned the word "collateral." He said I had good collaterals. I've only heard that term used in reference to banking.

When one of your main arteries becomes blocked, nature tries to compensate. Nature has an incredible wealth of techniques and options at her disposal to deal, at least initially and partially, with almost any abnormality with which she is faced. In the case of a blocked main artery, nature cannot usually restore that artery, but she can open up parallel smaller channels. Those smaller channels are known as "collateral" blood vessels. Although they are small, the collaterals can be multiple or numerous. They can often carry enough flow to prevent a heart attack. Sometimes, they can even carry adequate flow to eliminate angina. But collaterals take time to develop. So, in a slowly progressing blockage, the collaterals will also form slowly and progressively. A sudden severe blockage, nonetheless, will cause its damage before the minimum period of several days that collaterals require to open up and work.

These collaterals represent overgrowth of small capillary channels that are present normally but are called into action when the main blockage occurs. It is as if a detour route on a country road is opened by police when the main highway becomes blocked. The invocation of collateral blood vessels is yet another reflection of nature's infinite wisdom in dealing with medical abnormalities. Collaterals are depicted schematically in the accompanying figure.

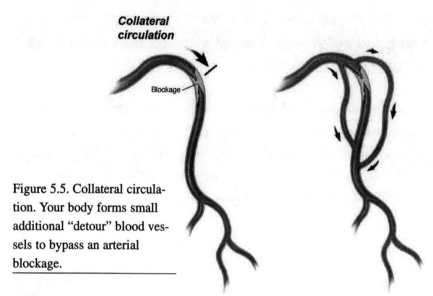

Figure 5.5. Collateral circulation. Your body forms small additional "detour" blood vessels to bypass an arterial blockage.

I have heard that a lot of people with coronary artery disease or heart attacks do not have high cholesterol. Can this be true?

You are entirely correct. At least half of all coronary artery disease patients do not have elevated cholesterol. Cholesterol is only part of the story. As discussed above, we really do not have all the answers to the reasons for arteriosclerosis. Smoking, poor diet, high blood pressure, and lack of exercise are additional factors. A positive family history for heart disease is also a serious risk factor. However, a considerable number of patients have none of these risk factors. This is the reason that there is room for alternate or supplementary theories, such as the infectious theory discussed previously in this chapter.

What can I do, practically speaking, to improve my heart's health and my well-being for the future?

Dr. Yusuf at the McMaster University in Toronto has identified nine specific measures each patient with heart disease can take to improve his or her future.[3] These measures also make sense for those who do not currently have heart disease but are anxious to prevent its development. These nine measures are linked directly to the nine most important risk factors leading to heart disease, which account for about 90 percent of the statistical risk for heart disease.

These measures are as follows:

1. **Control your cholesterol**. We cover the types of cholesterol and their importance elsewhere in this chapter. As a start, you need to know your cholesterol level. You can use diet, exercise, and drugs, if necessary, to bring a high cholesterol into line.

2. **Diabetes**. You need to avoid diabetes. Diabetes dramatically increases the frequency and severity of arteriosclerosis. To avoid diabetes, you should keep your weight down as you get older; this will help tremendously in avoiding late onset (Type II) diabetes. Regular exercise will help as well. If you already have diabetes, meticulously managing your sugar intake will help prevent arteriosclerosis.

3. **Control your stress**. Stress is an inherent part of life. Stress definitely contributes to coronary artery disease. We cannot eliminate stress from our lives. You should, however, take measures to control or eliminate recurrent sources of severe stress, either interpersonal or job-related.

4. **Obesity**. Obesity adds dramatically to your risk of heart disease and also contributes to high blood pressure and diabetes. Interestingly, recent studies have shown that it is

abdominal obesity—the area around your belly—in particular that is most dangerous. Keeping your weight in line
will help tremendously in keeping your heart and blood
vessels healthy.

5. **Cigarette smoking**. Smoking cigarettes is like rubbing the
   inside of your arteries with sandpaper. The inner lining is
   damaged, paving the way for cholesterol deposits to form.
   You simply must stop smoking. There are many aids for
   smoking cessation currently available through your pharmacy or general practitioner that can help you in this vital
   quest.

6. **High blood pressure**. High blood pressure damages your
   blood vessels, which leads to arteriosclerosis and heart disease. You must know your blood pressure. This will be
   measured in your doctor's office. You can also buy eco-
   nomical and accurate automatic blood pressure monitors at
   your pharmacy. If your blood pressure is high, work with
   your doctor to bring it in line, through weight reduction,
   diet, or medications. Your heart will thank you.

7. **Alcohol**. A drink a day is actually beneficial. Can you
   believe that? We are actually recommending to nonalco-
   holics that you have a drink a day, as do many families in
   Europe. Red wine is best, but other forms of alcohol are also
   helpful. We think this is because alcohol prevents platelets
   from becoming too sticky, thus clogging small vessels.
   However, if you consume more than a drink or two per day,
   you may promote heart failure or damage to your liver.

8. **Exercise**. Exercise is beneficial in every conceivable way.
   Exercise helps to keep your weight in check, decreases the
   likelihood of diabetes, drops your blood pressure, and preserves your muscle mass. You should partake in aerobic
   exercise (even walking suffices) at least five days a week.

9. **Diet**. Fruits and vegetables are the nutritional keys to heart health. They keep your cholesterol in check and cleanse damaging chemicals from around your cells.

So, here you have a list of specific measures you can take to avoid heart disease, or, if you already suffer from heart disease, to keep it in check.

10. We just wish you could follow step ten as well—*choose your parents carefully*! Heredity is the other key factor in your developing heart disease, and a very potent contributor at that. However, since you cannot really choose your parents, you should concentrate on steps one through nine.

Now for some follow-up on the patients detailed in this chapter:

Maria, the grandmother from Italy, whose hypertension caused a stroke, has just returned home from a rehab center. She is recovering the strength in the affected arm and leg. Her speech is almost normal. Her memory is still off, but it's improving. Her family sees to it that she takes her blood pressure medications religiously. They monitor her blood pressure four times a day with a home device.

Arnold Kramer, whose kidneys have failed from arteriosclerosis, has found that dialysis is not quite as bad as he anticipated. He tolerates the three-times-a-week sessions, albeit reluctantly, while he awaits a donor kidney organ.

The thirty-seven-year-old runner suffering from juvenile diabetes had her bypass operation. She did well for two years, at which time the diabetes began wreaking havoc on the vein grafts. She is stable on medications, but her future could be brighter. Another operation may be viable before she turns forty-five.

Mr. Amarante, the patient with diffuse arteriosclerosis, about whom the resident and your author were so concerned, did have his bypass operation. As feared, his kidneys did shut down—fortunately only for ten days. Subsequently, the kidneys resumed near baseline function. You will remember how concerned we were about the danger of a stroke from the operation. Our fears proved justified, as a stroke indeed occurred. It was a mild one, however, and Mr. A. has resumed an active life. It is only a matter of time until the arteriosclerotic disease in one vascular bed or another rears its ugly head, damaging his kidneys, brain, or heart.

Chapter
6
HEART ATTACKS

What should I do if I develop severe chest pain and feel quite ill?

Without question, 911 should be called and you should be brought to the nearest hospital. There are many reasons for this. More than half the patients who ultimately die of a heart attack do so within the first two hours after onset. They die of a cardiac arrhythmia, usually ventricular fibrillation. If this happens while the patient is at home, it is usually fatal. If it occurs in the emergency department of a hospital, it can almost always be reversed by the delivery of an electric shock to the chest—called *defibrillation.*

I hate the thought of going to a hospital if it may just be an upset stomach rather than my heart. Why not see if my pain will go away?

The most dangerous period after a heart attack is in the early minutes and the first several hours after it starts. That is because the risk of ventricular fibrillation (heart stoppage) is highest right after a heart attack, and diminishes as time passes. If ventricular fibrillation occurs outside the hospital, the likelihood of survival is slim. If it occurs within the hospital, it is almost always treatable. Therefore, although it is inconvenient to come to the emergency department if the problem turns out to be an upset stomach, it is a far better alternative to staying at home with an evolving early heart attack and risking sudden death. Besides the survival issues, you risk other difficulties and potential complications if you delay in going to the hospital.

If I go to the hospital with a heart attack, what are the doctors going to do?

The therapy for a patient who comes to the hospital with a heart attack has changed markedly over the years. A sequence of well-worked-out procedures will take place in an orderly manner. An intravenous line will be introduced into a vein in order to gain access to the circulation for the administration of medications. An electrocardiogram (EKG) will be taken to diagnose whether a heart attack has occurred. Blood will be drawn for diagnostic purposes to determine if there has been any heart damage. If there is evidence that a heart attack has occurred, lidocaine, an antiarrhythmic, will be given. A cardiac monitor will be applied to record the cardiac rhythms and ensure that no serious rhythm abnormalities occur. You will be administered oxygen to breathe, so that more oxygen can reach the aggrieved heart muscle cells. Morphine will be administered through an IV to make the pain of the heart attack subside. Doctors will decide whether a thrombolytic agent (a clot buster) should be given. Also, a decision will be made as to whether you should be brought to the cardiac catheterization laboratory to have a balloon angioplasty.

Medications to alter the effects of a heart attack will be administered. These include aspirin to help prevent a coronary clot from forming. A beta-blocker will likely be administered to cut down the work the heart has to do, and an ACE inhibitor may be given for much the same purpose.

Often, the patient will be given heparin, a powerful blood thinner, through IV. This can prevent further clot formation in the coronary artery.

There are a variety of thrombolytic medications known as *clot busters*. These medications actually dissolve clots in the coronary arteries. They go one giant step beyond heparin. Heparin prevents further clots from forming—a very good thing. The clot busters actually dissolve existing clots, an even more powerful effect. They are very strong and effective agents. They can result in complications, usually related to bleeding from unintended sites, such as the site of catheterization needlestick, the brain, or the back of the abdomen. Among commonly used thrombolytic medications are the following: t-PA, streptokinase, and urokinase. These drugs are only used within a four- to five-hour window after onset of chest pain and heart attack. If the heart muscle has been deprived of blood flow for longer than this, the heart attack zone is not going to be saved regardless of what drugs are given. Beyond this window of opportunity, the benefits of these powerful drugs do not justify the risks—particularly to the brain.

Alternatively, in hospitals where it is available, another form of therapy may be utilized. It is called Percutaneous Coronary Intervention (PCI) and may render even better results than thrombolytic therapy. The word *percutaneous* means "through the skin"—that is, without an incision. This entire procedure is done via a needlestick, usually in the large artery in the crease between the low abdomen and the thigh. In this form of therapy, a cardiac catheterization and coronary angiogram are performed on an emergency basis. Within the heart, the artery with the plaque and thrombus causing the heart attack are identified. Then, a balloon dilatation, or angioplasty, is performed—most often augmented by delivery of a metal stent (a fine metal scaffold designed to keep the artery from collapsing). The stent is placed along the inner surface of the artery by having the balloon expand, forcing the stent tightly against the arterial wall. The stents are metal with large gaps, similar to the struts of a child's erector set. Of late, the metal stents are coated with medication to help the artery to stay open. The results are immediate and dramatic: the offending artery is widened, ensuring adequate blood flow to the affected cardiac muscle.

How have medications altered the occurrence of a heart attack?

Medications have reduced the likelihood of occurrence of heart attacks and also altered the progression of a heart attack if it does occur. Aspirin has been shown to increase chances of survival if taken when a heart attack begins. Similarly, cholesterol-lowering drugs, particularly the statins, have decreased the incidence of heart attack.

If a heart attack does occur, a class of medications called thrombolytics may dissolve the offending coronary artery clot that is causing the heart attack. Although thrombolytics do not prevent a heart attack, they do decrease the severity of the event. As mentioned above, beta-blockers and ACE inhibitors also diminish the severity of the heart attack.

After you have recovered from the heart attack and for the long-term future, you will take two types of pills: beta-blockers to decrease your heart rate and ACE inhibitors to decrease your blood pressure and the workload on your heart.

What goes on in the CCU?

The coronary care unit (CCU) is a specialized unit where patients who have sustained a heart attack can be closely monitored and treated should there be any complication from the heart attack. Each patient's heart rhythm is separately monitored, and prophylactic (preventative) antiarrhythmic medication can be administered if necessary. Similarly, if the patient develops low blood pressure or congestive heart failure as a consequence of the heart attack, medications can be administered to help treat these complications. Generally speaking, coronary care units have an augmented nursing staff to help give the patient intensive nursing care. Experienced, specially trained physicians are on hand to cover the CCU at all times. Furthermore, it is very common for education programs on diet and lifestyle and physical rehabilitation training to begin in the coronary care unit, once your situation has stabilized.

Are the nurses empowered to provide emergency care if the doctor is away?

Time is often of great importance if a cardiac emergency occurs. This is particularly so if a life-threatening arrhythmia such as ventricular tachycardia or ventricular fibrillation occurs. Coronary care unit nurses are trained and have full responsibility for administering emergency care such as electrical defibrillation or intravenous medications to help combat rhythm or blood pressure problems.

When I came in, the doctor said my blood showed I had a heart attack; how can the blood show this?

If a heart attack is in progress, the affected heart muscle will start to die as a consequence of not receiving blood and oxygen. When that happens, intracellular enzymes will start to leak out of the heart muscle and into the blood. These enzymes are called troponins or

CKMB and are the mainstay of the enzymatic diagnosis of myocardial infarction. These abnormal blood enzymes, in conjunction with the EKG results and the patient's symptoms, determine whether or not a heart attack has occurred.

I heard my father's doctors talking on rounds about whether or not he suffered a "transmural" heart attack. What were they talking about?

You bring up a good question. The word *transmural* means "extending throughout the wall"—from *trans* for "through" and *mural* for "wall." A transmural heart attack is more extensive and more serious than a nontransmural heart attack.

A heart attack always starts on the inner surface of the heart, which we call the *endocardium*. The heart attack is like an iceberg, with the biggest part on the inner surface of the cardiac wall. As a heart attack becomes more extensive, it may involve the *myocardium*, the main muscle of the wall, and ultimately the *epicardium*, or outermost layer of the heart wall. The reason that heart attacks start on the inside of the wall is that the arteries run on the outer wall, on the surface of the heart. The inner part of the wall, the endocardium, is farthest away from the nutrient blood flow.

We can tell whether a heart attack is transmural or nontransmural from the EKG. A transmural heart attack produces a telltale signal on the EKG, which we call a Q-wave. For this reason, transmural infarctions are called Q-wave heart attacks, and nontransmural infarctions are called non–Q-wave heart attacks. In general, it is better to have a non–Q-wave than a Q-wave heart attack. If a patient is brought in promptly for care, the progression toward Q-wave heart attack can often be aborted by medical therapies, such as blood thinners, clot busters, nitroglycerine, and the like. In certain cases, angioplasty or even surgery may be applied to prevent this progression.

With a transmural heart attack, the entire involved wall dies, with little hope for rejuvenation by any therapies. With a nontransmural heart attack, there is hope for restoring some function, even later down the road, by angioplasty or coronary bypass surgery.

What is CPR?

Cardiopulmonary resuscitation is a rescue technique intended to replace the functions of breathing and circulation of blood in a patient whose heart has stopped.

While full instruction in cardiopulmonary resuscitation, or CPR, is beyond the scope of this book, we will provide an overview. Courses and formal instruction in CPR are available through your local community and through the American Heart Association. More and more of the general public are becoming trained in CPR. Dramatic rescues are seen daily because of this familiarity with resuscitation. Space in this book permits only brief discussion of key factors in CPR, which you will find immediately below.

How do I tell if a sick person needs CPR?

First and foremost you must determine whether the heart has stopped. If the patient is conscious, his heart has not stopped and he does not need CPR. The potential need for CPR arises only if the patient has suddenly become unconscious. Often the loss of consciousness has been witnessed by bystanders. If the person is indeed unconscious, your next step is to determine if he is breathing and if he has a pulse. In terms of breathing, you can check to see if his chest is rising and falling or if air is passing in and out of his nose or mouth. In terms of pulse, you can check at his wrist (radial pulse), at the groin crease (femoral pulse), or in the neck (carotid pulse). If you feel no pulse and see no regular breathing, then CPR is necessary.

How do I administer CPR?

To stimulate the beating of the heart, you must pump on the chest. If you compress the chest adequately, blood will flow forward to the body. The patient must be on a hard surface, on his back. It is not possible to perform effective cardiac compression on a soft surface. The floor is usually where the arrested patient finds himself, and this is an appropriate site for CPR. Your palms should go one over the other directly over the lower breastbone. You must press very hard—hard enough to make the breastbone nearly hit the spine. (You may break a rib or two, but that is a small price to pay for survival.) You will tire very quickly and it is best if someone can take over every few minutes. You should repeat the compressions rapidly, at least sixty to eighty times per minute.

Simultaneously, the lungs must be expanded, usually by mouth-to-mouth resuscitation. Special hygienic mouthpiece connectors may be available in some public places. Also, bellows bags attached to face masks, like pilots' masks, may be available, and may make you feel more comfortable. In the case of a loved one or a family member, you will probably not be uncomfortable giving direct mouth-to-mouth resuscitation. You should deliver eight to ten deep breaths per minute.

Can one person alone administer CPR?

Effective CPR can only be done by a single person if that person is trained and working under special circumstances. One of our colleagues singlehandedly performed CPR, both pumping and breathing, and called 911 as well, when his wife had a cardiac arrest from a sudden heart attack and they were both home alone. She is alive and well due specifically to his heroic efforts. In most settings, however, it will be very hard for you to do both cardiac compression and artificial respiration. At least two resuscitators are generally required. In most cases, another person will be available to help, and one person can do compression while the other does the breathing.

In many cases, especially in malls, on airplanes, or in other public places, a doctor, nurse, firefighter, police officer, or paramedic will arrive to assist your efforts. But often it is the quick action of a member of the general public that has saved the life of a person with a sudden cardiac arrest.

If someone in your family has heart disease, you may find that this gives you an extra incentive to pursue training in CPR, so that you can be ready to meet a potential emergency.

Are there any technical devices available in public places to help a layperson administer CPR?

In more and more public places, automatic defibrillators are available. These devices are like the paddles that you have seen used on medical television shows. For the models in public places, the paddles are coupled with a smart medical computer. When you place the paddles on the chest of an unconscious person, the computer determines if the patient has ventricular fibrillation—the chaotic cardiac rhythm that causes a cardiac arrest. If the machine detects this rhythm, it automatically fires a DC current. In many cases, early application of this electric current will restore a heartbeat and terminate the arrest. If the patient starts to breathe, if you feel a pulse, and if consciousness is restored, your efforts have been successful.

How about home defibrillators?

In fact, home defibrillators have now become quite widespread. They can be purchased for just over $1,000. If your family can afford one, you should buy a home defibrillator. Having this foresight can literally save a life, especially given the long delays that may occur before the arrival of emergency personnel after a 911 call. Often, resuscitative efforts are useless if the arrival of the ambulance is delayed. With a home defibrillator, you can restore a rhythm and consciousness on your own—at the best possible time: right after the cardiac arrest has occurred.

TESTS AND DIAGNOSES

THE PHYSICAL EXAM

What does the doctor check when he examines my heart?

There is considerable information that the doctor can learn by examining the heart. First, the heart rate—the number of times per minute that the heart beats—can be determined. Whether the heart is beating slower or faster than optimal can be a clue to an underlying problem. The stethoscope is used to hear a noise called a murmur. These noises come from blood flow through a narrowed valve, or blood flow through a leaky valve. Certain rhythm disturbances can be diagnosed by the use of the stethoscope. Cardiac extra beats, dropped beats, or a totally irregular rhythm (atrial fibrillation) can be diagnosed. Finally, in hearts that are weakened in their pumping abilities, subtle sounds called gallops can be heard, which gives the physician insights into how to most effectively treat a patient.

The accompanying diagram shows the areas where we commonly listen to the heart tones and indicates which valves are heard best in which territory.

In addition to examining your heart, the doctor will also check other parts of your body that give information about your heart. If

Areas of ausculation

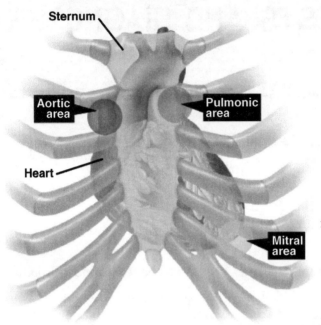

Figure 7.1. Sites of common murmurs. *Ausculation* is the medical term for listening, so this figure shows where the physician listens for the different murmurs that can affect the heart.

he hears "rales," or "wet" sounds when he listens to your lungs, that implies excess pressure in your heart and lungs, from valve disease or heart failure. If your doctor sees edema fluid at your ankles, that again signifies backup of fluids at the heart level—further evidence of heart failure.

Also, your doctor will inspect the veins at your neck. If these veins are excessively full, that implies elevated pressure in your heart, indicating heart failure. We check the fullness of these veins as we gradually raise the back of the examining table, sitting you up more and more fully. The veins should become nearly flat by an elevation of thirty to forty-five degrees.

You can estimate the pressure in your heart yourself, by a simple test. Sit in a chair without sides in the center of your room, so that you have the space to raise your arms at your sides. Start with your arms at your sides, hanging toward the floor. Note that the veins in the backs of your hands are full, indicating that they are pressurized. Now, slowly raise your arms perpendicular to your body, as if you were doing a slow jumping jack. The veins should become flat by the time your arms reach heart level, or certainly by shoulder level. If the veins are still full by the time your arms are at the level of your ears or the top of your head, then the pressure in your heart is too high.

This test uses gravity, rather than a sophisticated medical apparatus, to assess the venous pressures in your heart. The point is that the pressure in your right atrium is transmitted to the veins in your hands. If the right atrial pressure is too high, the veins in your hands will stay full as you raise your arms perpendicularly.

The accompanying figure will help you to perform this simple test.

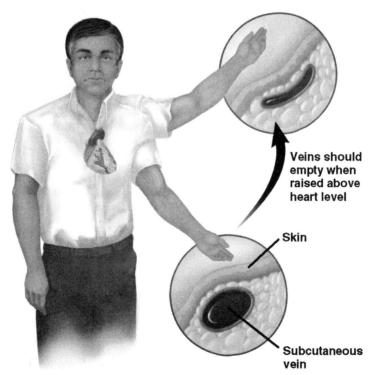

Veins should empty when raised above heart level

Skin

Subcutaneous vein

Figure 7.2. Estimating the pressure in your heart.

My doctor says I have a heart murmur. What is a heart murmur?

The heart has four valves, two on the right side of the heart and two on the left side of the heart. The right-sided valves are named the tricuspid valve and the pulmonary valve. The left-sided valves are named the mitral valve and the aortic valve.

Normally these valves open and close rhythmically, allowing blood alternately to enter a heart chamber and to be ejected from it. When valves are neither narrowed nor leaky, this process occurs silently. Blood flows smoothly through a normal-sized valve and does not leak backward if the valve closes normally.

However, if a valve is narrowed (or *stenotic*) the blood moving forward becomes turbulent—as if a wide river is forced to progress through a narrowing between its banks. The site of the flowing river through a narrowed part is called a rapid, where, as you know, the usually quietly flowing river becomes a noisy one.

If a valve is leaky, it is termed *regurgitant*. If the tricuspid valve is leaky, when the right ventricle contracts, blood will flow backward through this leaky valve, mixing with blood entering the right atrium from the great veins. If the mitral valve is leaky, when the left ventricle contracts, blood will flow backward through the leaky valve, mixing with blood entering the left atrium from the pulmonary veins. This causes turbulence, and a murmur occurs.

We grade heart murmurs on a scale of I to VI. A grade I murmur can be heard only by an expert cardiologist. A grade II murmur can be heard by most physicians. A grade III murmur can be heard by medical students. Grade IV and V murmurs are very loud. A grade VI murmur can be heard even with the stethoscope off the chest wall.

If a murmur is especially loud, it can produce what we call a *thrill*. A thrill refers to a vibration that can be felt by a hand placed

over the heart. To have a thrill, a patient must have extremely turbulent flow across his valve. Invariably, there is a high-grade
murmur associated with a thrill.

Is every murmur significant?

No. Some murmurs are called *functional* (or *innocent*) murmurs,
occurring even in the presence of a normal valve, and some are
called *organic*, reflecting an abnormality of the valve. At times
blood may flow so rapidly through even a normal-sized valve that a
murmur occurs. But the determination of whether a murmur is functional or organic should be made by your physician. An echocardiogram or ultrasound will sometimes be ordered to help determine if
the murmur is innocent or due to an abnormality of the valve.

EKG

What can you tell from a simple EKG?

Although the EKG (electrocardiogram) is a simple, inexpensive
test that has been utilized since the turn of the century, it does provide a great deal of information about your heart—both its current
status and its history.

The contraction of your heart muscle is brought about through
electrical stimulation, which originates in the heart's natural pacemaking tissue. The "clock" that drives your heartbeat is the sinus
node in the right atrium, one of the upper chambers of the heart.
The impulse then travels through a "connecting station" called the
A-V node, located between the atria and the ventricles. From there,
the electrical impulse travels down very fine, intricately arranged

electrical fibers into the powerful lower chambers of the heart, the ventricles. See figure 7.3a.

These minute electrical signals are amplified by the internal apparatus of the EKG machine into signals that are recorded on printed paper. The EKG machine "looks" at your heart from twelve different angles, hence the twelve leads of a standard EKG.

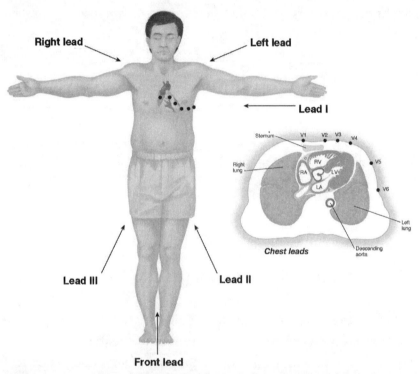

Figures 7.3a and 7.3b. The twelve leads through which the EKG "looks" at your heart. Six "limb" leads are seen in figure a and six "chest" leads in figure b.

Do not try to interpret the EKG yourself. This will lead to unnecessary concern. The EKG traces are nearly indecipherable without extensive training. Even our best students find EKG interpretation extremely demanding. Your EKG, should you see it, will probably look extremely bizarre and possibly worrisome. Let your doctor interpret the EKG for you.

The EKG signal recordings reveal a tremendous amount of information about your heart and its history. First, they characterize the rhythm of your heart (see the section titled "Arrhythmias" in chapter 3).

Second, the electrical signals indicate whether your heart is suffering from inadequate blood flow at the present time. In such a case, one finds electrical evidence of *ischemia*, which means inadequate blood flow. Ischemia can be regional, affecting only certain zones of your heart muscle. Ischemia is manifested by inversion of the T-waves of your EKG. The T-waves are the last blips in the EKG signal of a heartbeat. As can be seen in figure 7.4, the T-waves are like the "tail" of the EKG trace.

Third, the EKG indicates whether there is any actual injury in

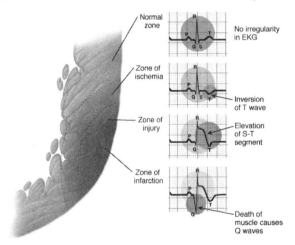

Figure 7.4. EKG examples of ischemia, injury, and infarction (death) of cardiac muscle.

progress to your heart muscle at the present time. Injury or death of heart muscle fibers is the result of prolonged inadequate blood flow, or ischemia.

Finally, the EKG shows whether you have suffered a heart attack in the past. An old heart attack is manifested by loss of electrical forces from the corresponding zone of the heart muscle. This is technically referred to as onset of Q-waves, or downward deflection of the line of the EKG, in contradistinction to the normal upward deflection from a certain zone.

Thus, this simple, painless, risk-free test provides your doctor a tremendous amount of valuable information concerning the current status of your heart and its past history.

THE STRESS TEST

What is a stress test?

If your doctor suspects that you may have blocked coronary arteries, he will likely send you for a stress test. This is also called an exercise test. The aim is to see if exercise can provoke symptoms and signs indicative of coronary artery disease.

The exercise is usually administered by having you walk on a treadmill. The speed and inclination of the treadmill are increased gradually over the duration of the test.

The first indication the doctor looks for is whether you feel chest pain during the test. If you feel pain as your level of exertion increases, then you are quite likely having insufficient blood flow to your heart—which indicates coronary artery disease.

However, at least one-third to one-half of patients do not feel heart pain in the normal way. Diabetic patients are especially likely not to feel cardiac pain. So, the doctor will look for other clues.

If your blood pressure drops as your exertion increases, that is a bad sign. That indicates that your heart is not receiving sufficient blood flow for the work it has to perform. A drop in blood pressure is one of the most serious indicators from a stress test.

The doctor will also check your EKG continuously as you exercise. If your heart is not receiving sufficient blood flow, certain characteristic changes occur in your EKG tracing, even if you do not feel pain. These changes can indicate that your exercise test is positive for coronary artery disease.

Under stress, you may develop abnormal heartbeats or rhythms. These add evidence of insufficient blood flow to your heart.

To increase the sensitivity of the exercise test even more, your doctor will probably combine the test with ECHO (echocardiogram) or nuclear images of your heart. These tests can provide objective, scientific evidence that your heart is not receiving sufficient blood flow during exercise. For example, if, under stress, one zone of your heart shows less radioisotope uptake, that indicates insufficient blood flow to that region.

The stress test is a very good screening investigation for blocked arteries to the heart muscle. If the test is negative, chances are very good that your arteries are clean and your heart is not the source of your symptoms. Likewise, if the test is positive, chances are very high that you have real coronary artery disease.

What will the stress test feel like to me?

If it is a regular stress test, done with ordinary exercise, you will feel like you are having an aerobic workout at the gym. You will walk on a treadmill at an increasing pace or angle until you complete the entire protocol (rare) or until you experience chest pain or severe shortness of breath. The test may also be terminated by the doctor if he sees worrisome abnormalities on your EKG. The entire exercise will not take longer than fifteen minutes.

If your test is being supplemented by nuclear images, you will have an IV injection before starting the test.

If you are unable to walk for the stress component, you may be given one of a number of drugs that stress your heart. You may feel warmth or flushing or even light-headedness from the medication.

Please remember that, unlike a school test, you cannot "do better" by studying or willing yourself on your cardiac exercise test. Either you have or do not have blockages. If you do, they have likely built up over decades. You cannot influence this process on the morning of your stress test. All we ask is that you do your best to comply with instructions, be willing to walk long enough and hard enough so that adequate information is obtained, and keep the doctor and technician apprised of everything that you are feeling.

But if you suspect I have coronary artery disease, how can you subject me to the trauma of an exercise test? Will I be safe?

Although we will be stressing your heart, you will be very well monitored and extremely safe. There will be a technician and a doctor in constant attendance. The test will be terminated as soon as any worrisome changes are noted. In case of any adverse event, immediate treatment can be administered. The chance of any serious complication from your stress test is extremely remote.

THE CATHETERIZATION

The doctor said that I need to have a cardiac catheterization. What is that?

The cardiac catheterization is the gold standard approach to getting to know your heart. It is performed by passing fine wires and tubes into your heart, usually through the large arteries and veins in your groin.

First, the doctor will use a fine tube to measure the pressures

You will remember the case described in chapter 1 of Robert, the telephone worker who was stricken with chest pain while he was repairing a phone line high above the ground. You will recall that his partner got him to the emergency room and from there he was transferred to the CCU with a diagnosis of impending heart attack. In fact, he underwent a cardiac catheterization. This showed severe three-vessel disease (blockages in all three major coronary arteries) as well as a left main lesion (a blockage in the main arterial trunk that supplies the heart). Surgery was recommended. Robert and his family were considering the recommendation. There seemed to be no other choice.

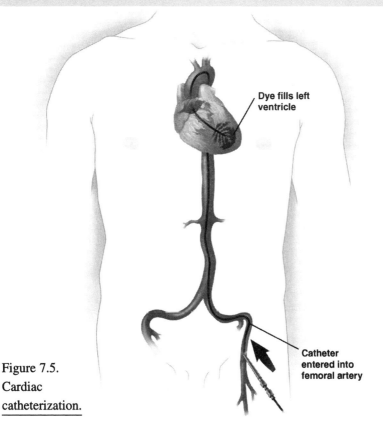

Dye fills left
ventricle

Catheter
entered into
femoral artery

Figure 7.5.
Cardiac
catheterization.

inside your heart and lungs. In general, it is better to have low pressures in the cardiac chambers and lungs, as this indicates that blood is flowing forward without impediment. The pressure measurements can also give an indication about whether you have any narrowed heart valves, specifically aortic stenosis or mitral stenosis.

Second, the doctor will inject dye into the chambers of your heart—usually into the left ventricle and occasionally into the aorta. This injection of dye allows the doctor to make your heart chambers visible, so that the pattern and strength of contraction can be assessed. Also, any abnormal flow patterns, like leaky valves from aortic regurgitation or mitral regurgitation, can be detected.

Finally, the doctor will inject dye into the coronary arteries themselves, providing the ultimate means of visualizing any blockages. This is important in patients with angina or heart attack. This method of assessing the coronary arteries far surpasses any other indirect means, such as a stress test, a thallium test, or the like. (Thallium is a nuclear tracer [albeit a safe one!] that can be used to visualize blood flow in a "nuclear" stress test.)

What will the experience of catheterization be like from my perspective?

The catheterization will not be nearly as bad as you might expect. The entire process usually takes less than one hour. You will be premedicated with a sedative drug before going to the laboratory, so that you will already be pleasantly calm on arrival. You will be draped so that the groin area is exposed. (As explained previously, some cardiologists, however, use the elbow or wrist.) That area will be washed thoroughly with antiseptic. You will feel a small needlestick as the doctor "cannulates" the vessels; that medical term means to place a fine tube into the artery and vein. The remainder of the process is painless. Depending on your wishes, you can even watch the catheters dance around your cardiac chambers on a small X-ray screen. Some patients wouldn't miss this show for the world; others want no part of it whatsoever. You may feel a warm, flushed sensation when the large aliquot (volume) of dye is injected during certain parts of the procedure. Sometimes that sensation can be a bit frightening. Just by being forewarned—as you are now by reading this—your fear can be alleviated considerably.

Chances are that, like most of our patients, you will say afterward that the worst part of the catheterization was lying on a cold, hard table and getting a backache.

Will the catheterization be painful?

Surprisingly, this test is not usually painful. The needlestick is about the same as when you have your blood drawn. Amazingly, the inner surfaces of the blood vessels and the inner surface of the heart, which are traversed by the fine wires and tubes, have no nerve endings for pain. You will not—in fact, you *can*not—feel the wires and tubes as they make their progress and do their important work.

Is a catheterization dangerous?

In fact, catheterization is extremely safe. Death from catheterization is almost unheard of in the current day, occurring at less than one in a thousand procedures. Perforation of the heart is very rare. Very, very rarely, one of the coronary arteries can be injured so that it splits internally and requires a bypass operation. Almost without exception, catheterization is quick, comfortable, and extremely informative.

The dye used in catheterization can occasionally produce an

allergic reaction. The dye is usually based on iodine, so if you have a fish allergy, you should let your doctor know. If you have had prior allergic reactions to medical dye, it is imperative that you make your catheterization team aware.

Rarely, the dye used for catheterization can produce a decrease in your kidney function. This is usually transient. New techniques have decreased the chance of this occurring. This does not usually occur unless you have some preexisting kidney disease.

One of my friends had his catheterization done through his arm. Can I have that too?

Sometimes, the leg arteries have their own blockages, so they do not provide free access to your heart. The fine tubes and wires simply cannot pass through the blocked portions. In such a case, your cardiologist may pass the wires through your arm, either at the elbow or at the armpit area. There are relatively large arteries and veins at these locations, as in your groin, which lead to the heart. These are not commonly affected by arteriosclerosis or blockages.

In some cases, cardiologists prefer the arm over the groin for catheterization, even in patients whose leg arteries are open and would provide a direct route to the heart. The arm approach can be less uncomfortable and allow quicker mobility after the test is done. In some cases, the cardiologist may use miniaturized wires and tubes and place them through the even smaller artery at your wrist. Recovery is especially quick with this approach.

Do I need to be admitted to the hospital for my catheterization?

In the present day, for stable patients coming from home, catheterization is almost always done on an outpatient basis. You come in during the morning and are home by day's end, after a period of observation in a recovery room. You can be back to your normal activities within just a few days.

I heard on TV that catheterization is no longer necessary. I can have a simple MRI instead. Is this true?

To find a noninvasive means to visualize the coronary arteries has been like the holy grail for cardiology. It is true that advanced CT scans and MRI (magnetic resonance imaging) scans can give glimpses of the coronary arteries. At this time, despite manufacturers' hype, no technology other than catheterization provides exact, reliable, detailed information about your coronary arteries and their blockages. Perhaps in the future, the alternate scans, which can be done without tubes and wires, will reach fruition. We are not there yet.

At the very moment that this book is being published, a new generation of CT scanners (the so-called sixty-four-slice machines) are sweeping the nation. The images from these advanced machines are truly extraordinary. The potential for replacing catheterization with this less-invasive modality appears on the verge of being realized. Formal comparative studies are under way, and clinicians everywhere are "testing the waters," so to speak, by ordering high-tech CT scans in place of catheterizations.

OTHER TESTS

My doctor is sending me for an ECHO test. What is that?

The echocardiogram—also abbreviated "echo" or "ECHO," is an extremely valuable and noninvasive way to glean a tremendous amount of information about your heart. By noninvasive, we mean without needle punctures or incisions, and without discomfort. The echo test uses sound waves that are passed into your chest toward your heart. The reflection of these sound waves produces dramatic pictures of your heart in action—like a real-time action cam. It shows your heart chambers, your valves, and your aorta.

Echo is remarkably benign. We even use the test on babies and on the unborn fetus, as most modern mothers know. As far as we can tell, the echo test is entirely harmless. It is also quite a comfortable test. An echo jelly is spread on your chest and the probe is gently rubbed along your skin, almost like a massage.

Valve diseases—like aortic stenosis/regurgitation or mitral stenosis/regurgitation—are reliably detected by echo. In fact, echo is the optimal method to visualize valves in live action—even better than looking directly at the valves in the operating room. In the operating room, to see a valve directly, the heart must be stopped so that the chambers can be open. Although we can see the valves directly, they are no longer "in action" at this point.

Also, the echo shows us the pumping strength, or ejection fraction, of your heart. In this way, we learn whether you have suffered prior heart damage, and, if so, its extent.

Is there anything the echo doesn't show?

Yes, the echo cannot show us the coronary arteries or blockages in those arteries. They are simply too small to be seen without catheterization.

However, by showing function of various portions of your heart under exercise, the echo can be an important part of a stress test. In this way, the echo provides indirect information about potential blocked coronary arteries.

I had an echo. Now my doctor wants to do something called a *TEE.* I didn't like the sound of that. Is this test really necessary?

The ordinary echo, done through the skin of your chest, is called a *TTE*, or *transthoracic* echo. This is painless. However, this approach has some limitations. Remember that much of your heart is surrounded by your lungs. Your lungs contain air, and air does not transmit the sound waves of the echo machine well.

There is a way to get echo access to your heart with no intervening air. Your esophagus, your swallowing tube, passes directly behind your heart. By passing a scope containing an echo probe through your mouth and down your esophagus, your doctor can obtain incredibly precise and detailed echo images of your heart. Because this test is done via your esophagus, it is called a TEE, for transesophageal echocardiogram. When fine details of anatomy are required, this is the approach of choice. It can be uncomfortable to swallow the echo probe, but with mild sedation, most patients find this not terribly objectionable. Usually, the results are well worth the temporary discomfort.

NUCLEAR IMAGING

I don't like the sound of a "nuclear" test of my heart. Is it dangerous? Why would I need it?

Your heart can be visualized by what we call *nuclear* means. A small aliquot of your blood is harvested and rendered very mildly radioactive. It is reinfused through your vein. Then, a nuclear camera uses the mildly radioactive blood as a "dye" to take pictures of your heart.

Because the camera is so powerful and magnifies the minute amount of radioactivity so powerfully, the amount of radiation to which you are exposed is extremely small. Hence, the test is very, very safe. There is no discomfort beyond having your blood drawn.

The nuclear technique can image the size and pumping strength of your heart in a test called a *MUGA* or an *ERNA* scan. This provides a precise, numerical, reproducible assessment of your ejection fraction, or the pumping strength of your heart. Many feel this is now the gold standard for assessing the strength of the heart, surpassing even catheterization for this particular assessment.

Nuclear images are often combined as part of your stress test. The nuclear camera can follow the flow of radioactive blood through your heart muscle, pinpointing regions that are deprived of blood because of blockages in the coronary arteries.

What is a normal "ejection fraction"? Shouldn't mine be 100 percent?

The ejection fraction is the percentage of blood leaving the heart with each beat, or contraction, compared with how much blood was there just before the contraction began. For example, if the left ventricle contains 100 millileters of blood at the moment it starts to contract, and it pumps 70 millileters of blood out to the body, then the left ventricular ejection fraction is 70 percent. If the left ventricle contains 200 millileters of blood just before the contraction, and ejects 140 millileters, the ejection fraction would still be 70 percent. The normal ejection fraction is in the 70 percent range. Since the left ventricle never empties completely, it is not possible (nor necessarily advantageous) to have an ejection fraction of 100 percent. If the heart-pumping qualities are damaged, the ejection fraction will diminish. Symptoms generally will not occur until the ejection fraction falls below 40 percent.

What can a CAT scan tell you about my heart?

We usually obtain a CAT scan, or CT scan, of your heart if we are concerned about a tumor in or around your heart. This is usually the type of tumor called a cardiac myxoma.

CAT scans of the heart are being offered by entrepreneurial outfits as screening tools for coronary artery disease. These particular scans are known by the names Electron Beam CT and Ultrafast CT. These scans report the amount of calcium in and around your coronary arteries, on a scale of 0 to 400. As insurers do not pay for these screening tests, they are obtained at your request and at your expense. These scans can also pick up asymptomatic tumors in different parts of your body. The clinical usefulness and proper role of such screening CT scans remains to be determined. The screening technique is eerily reminiscent of the TV show *Star Trek*, in which Dr. "Bones" McCoy would pass a scanning probe over every patient's body, giving him all the information that he needed to know, without his ever laying a hand on the patient himself.

What can an MRI scan tell you about my heart?

MRI, or magnetic resonance imaging, scans are like CAT scans, in that a machine takes computer-enhanced images of your body—in this case, your heart.

An MRI provides incredibly vivid moving pictures of your heart in action, showing details of your chambers, valves, and blood flow. These real-time moving pictures are beautiful to watch. And they are noninvasive and easy to obtain.

Although the pictures of your heart are beautiful, we do not yet have a general application for their use in cardiac patients. This is currently an extremely powerful technology seeking an appropriate application.

Of course, both CAT scans and MRIs are extremely useful in many other areas and are applied clinically every day to visualize not your heart per se, but rather the aorta, the main artery that begins from your heart and supplies all the organs of your body.

What will the MRI feel like?

Although this test is painless and requires only that you lie still, some patients find being enclosed in the tubelike apparatus of the MRI to be anxiety provoking. If you think you might feel this way, ask your doctor to prescribe a mild sedative prior to the test. Patients may also be bothered by the loud thumping or "hammering" noise that emanates from the machine. You may want to ask if you can bring earplugs or if earplugs can be provided. The tests usually take between fifteen and thirty minutes.

Chapter

8

LIVING WITH HEART DISEASE: LIFESTYLE CHANGES THAT PROTECT YOUR HEART

What can I eat?

Every day, in newspapers or magazines or on television or radio, you are given information about what some recent study showed about what to eat and what not to eat. All this information can be very confusing.

In general, if you have arteriosclerosis or coronary artery disease, or if your cholesterol or triglyceride levels are elevated, you should limit the amount of fat in your diet. Many excellent resources are available to guide you in tailoring your diet. A rough guide is to eat less cheese and butter and to eat red meat no more than twice a week.

Please remember that you do not need to impair your quality of life by making your diet too strict. The impact of diet on progression of arteriosclerosis, while beneficial, is not overwhelming. Also, remember that everyone needs to eat *something*. If we followed every latest article or advisory in the media (often based only on animal studies, which may or may not be relevant to humans), no one would be allowed to eat anything.

How about salt?

Patients with high blood pressure should use salt sparingly, but most patients with coronary artery disease do not have to be particularly concerned about their salt intake. If, however, the patient with coronary artery disease has congestive heart failure, then salt restriction is necessary.

Do I really need to stop smoking?

Yes, you absolutely, positively need to stop smoking. Smoking damages your arteries immensely. Your chance of restoring cardiac health nearly vanishes—no matter what treatments, medications, or operations are applied—if you continue to smoke. Get help from your general practitioner or internist. She can help you kick this habit that is literally killing you.

How can I bring my blood pressure back down to normal?

Lifestyle changes are important, and there is much that a person can do in order to bring blood pressure back down to normal. These lifestyle changes relate to (1) moderation in the use of salt in foods, (2) achieving an optimal weight (a body mass index of 25–26), and (3) a regular exercise program. To the extent that stress can be eliminated from the daily routine, that is desirable. These lifestyle changes are sometimes sufficient to control high blood pressure, but medication must at times be added in order to ensure a normal blood pressure around the clock.

   Body mass index (or BMI) compares your weight to your height.[1] Of course, taller individuals should normally weigh more,

Determining your Body Mass Index (BMI)

To use the table, find the appropriate height in the left-hand column. Move across the row to the given weight. The number at the top of the colum is the BMI for that height and weight.

BMI (kg/m²)	19	20	21	22	23	24	25	26	27	28	29	30	35	40
Height (in.)	Weight (lb.)													
58	91	96	100	105	110	115	119	124	129	134	138	143	167	191
59	94	99	104	109	114	119	124	128	133	138	143	148	173	198
60	97	102	107	112	118	123	128	133	138	143	148	153	179	204
61	100	106	111	116	122	127	132	137	143	148	153	158	185	211
62	104	109	115	120	126	131	136	142	147	153	158	164	191	218
63	107	113	118	124	130	135	141	146	152	158	163	169	197	225
64	110	116	122	128	134	140	145	151	157	163	169	174	204	232
65	114	120	126	132	138	144	150	156	162	168	174	180	210	240
66	118	124	130	136	142	148	155	161	167	173	179	186	216	247
67	121	127	134	140	146	153	159	166	172	178	185	191	223	255
68	125	131	138	144	151	158	164	171	177	184	190	197	230	262
69	128	135	142	149	155	162	169	176	182	189	196	203	236	270
70	132	139	146	153	160	167	174	181	188	195	202	207	243	278
71	136	143	150	157	165	172	179	186	193	200	208	215	250	286
72	140	147	154	162	169	177	184	191	199	206	213	221	258	294
73	144	151	159	166	174	182	189	197	204	212	219	227	265	302
74	148	155	163	171	179	186	194	202	210	218	225	233	272	311
75	152	160	168	176	184	192	200	208	216	224	232	240	279	319
76	156	164	172	180	189	197	205	213	221	230	238	246	287	328

Risk of Associated Disease According to BMI and Waist Size		Waist less than or equal to 40 in. (men) or 35 in. (women)	Waist greater than 40 in. (men) or 35 in. (women)
BMI			
18.5 or less	Underweight	--	N/A
18.5 - 24.9	Normal	--	N/A
25.0 - 29.9	Overweight	Increased	High
30.0 - 34.9	Obese	High	Very High
35.0 - 39.9	Obese	Very High	Very High
40 or greater	Extremely Obese	Extremely High	Extremely High

Figure 8.1. Calculation of body mass index.

and this criterion, the body mass index, takes that relationship into account. You can calculate your body mass index by dividing your weight in pounds by your height in inches, with the conversion factor shown in the equation below

$$\text{Body Mass Index (BMI)} = 705 \times \frac{\text{weight (pounds)}}{\text{height (inches)}^2}$$

You can also use the chart on the previous page to plot your BMI. Simply connect lines representing your weight with your height. The point of intersection corresponds to the indicated zones of BMI at the top of the chart.

You should aim to get your body mass index into the range of 25 to 26. Of course, as we approach or exceed middle age, some increase in weight is almost inevitable, so a measure of leniency in expected BMI is warranted.

Can I continue to have a drink with dinner?

Yes. There is no reason why you should not have a drink each evening with your dinner. As mentioned previously in this book, unless you are an alcoholic, wine with dinner may even help keep your heart free from coronary artery disease. Of course, moderation is essential. Excess consumption of alcohol is deleterious to both your heart and your liver, as well as other organs.

We've sometimes used cocaine at parties. It's not that dangerous, is it?

If you use cocaine, be afraid for your heart, very afraid. Cocaine has many actions pertinent to your heart—all of them bad. Cocaine increases your pulse and blood pressure, at times drastically. That in itself increases the load on your heart. The blood pressure increase can be so great that your aorta, the main artery of your body, fractures internally, causing a fatal condition known as an aortic dissection. Cocaine can cause life-threatening arrhythmias. Cocaine can constrict your coronary arteries so severely that you can suffer a major heart attack—even if you have no underlying arteriosclerotic coronary artery blockages.

And don't think that you can only get in trouble if you use this drug regularly. Occasional and even first-time users can also fall victim to these devastating effects.

What is the role of exercise in preventing heart disease?

Exercise is beneficial in a number of ways. The heart is a muscle and, like any other muscle in the body, it becomes more efficient when used. A well-conditioned athlete generally has a slow heart rate, as his heart is able to pump out more blood with each beat. Further, the other muscles of the body become more efficient with exercise and therefore extract oxygen more effectively from the blood that is pumped to them. Thus, the heart does not have to pump as much blood each minute. Exercise generally is useful in lowering blood pressure, as the small blood vessels of the body dilate or relax after the period of exercise is over. You can expect a drop in pressure of 10 millimeters of mercury (mmHg). Ancillary benefits reside in the fact that exercise burns calories and is a useful adjunct to weight reduction. Furthermore, exercise will raise your level of HDL, the good cholesterol, by about 10 percent. If you are a diabetic, exercise will lower your blood glucose levels by using up sugar and also by making your body more sensitive to its own insulin. Also, an individual who exercises regularly will generally not be a smoker, thereby eradicating a potent risk factor to the development of coronary artery disease.

What vitamins should I take to prevent or discourage heart disease?

It is hard to say with authority which vitamins are reasonable to take to discourage heart disease. Definitive research on this topic is very complex to attain, as so many factors enter into determining cardiac risk. Also, you have likely noticed from various news and media sources that recommendations tend to change like the wind from year to year, in accordance with the most recent reports. We can, however, make the following general points.

The vitamin niacin, one of the B-complex group, can reduce bad cholesterol, especially the worst subtypes, as well as triglycerides. Niacin can be dangerous, however, and you should consult with your doctor before starting a specific niacin program.

Folic acid, or folate, helps to lower your homocysteine levels.

Vitamin C is thought to be an important antioxidant. Antioxidant compounds prevent the adverse cellular changes resulting from wear and tear of metabolic processes. Vitamin E is thought to act similarly.

While we cannot prove that these vitamins will prevent your heart disease, it is a reasonable bet at this point in our medical understanding that they do protect your heart to some extent. However, megadoses are dangerous.

Although these antioxidant vitamins make theoretical sense, a recently released controlled study failed to show benefit from even a cocktail of several antioxidant vitamins.

Most multivitamin tablets contain at least some measure of these vitamins. You should ask your doctor about taking supplemental doses.

How about my diabetes? Do I need to control that to improve the outlook for my heart?

By all mean, yes, you need to control your diabetes to prevent rapid progression of coronary artery disease and arteriosclerosis. Diabetes causes especially severe coronary artery disease that tends to narrow the entire artery from top to bottom. For nondiabetics, the narrowing tends to be more localized. In diabetics, even the small branches are often diseased, which makes it difficult to find a spot to place a graft during the coronary artery bypass procedure.

What you can do is keep your preprandial (before meals) blood sugars and your bedtime blood sugars around the value of 100 milligrams per deciliter.

What is the effect of exercise on whether or not I develop a coronary artery disease problem?

Regular aerobic exercise (walking, jogging, swimming) is generally useful in helping to prevent heart disease. Exercise is beneficial in several ways. In general, LDL cholesterol will be modestly lowered by exercise and HDL cholesterol will rise. These are *good* changes. Patients who exercise generally have an easier time maintaining an optimal weight. Further, it is likely that regular exercise helps to develop coronary artery collateral vessels if there should be areas of narrowing in the coronary artery system. Therefore, if a blockage does develop in a coronary artery, the act of exercising will likely have generated auxiliary blood vessels that can be called into action.

Jim Fixx was a marathon runner, yet he died with severe coronary artery disease. How could this happen?

Exercise is only one of the factors that have an impact on whether or not coronary artery disease may develop. Jim Fixx was an extremely well-trained athlete, but he grew up in a time in which high blood pressure or high cholesterol could not be effectively treated. Also, exercise alone, although beneficial, cannot completely negate the impact of the other risk factors we have discussed. The fact that he could run marathons in spite of having severe coronary artery disease is a testimony to how well conditioned he was. It is always possible that he would have died even earlier were he not such a superbly trained athlete.

I have diabetes. Does that mean I will definitely develop a coronary artery problem?

Having diabetes certainly will predispose you to developing coronary artery disease, as well as other manifestations of arteriosclerosis. However, there is much that you can do to minimize this risk.

Diabetes mellitus may be Type 1 or Type 2. Type 1 diabetes tends to occur earlier in life and requires insulin therapy. It will not respond to oral medications.

Type 2 diabetes is susceptible to oral medication, at least for some period of time. Over the past decades there have been a number of agents developed to treat the patient with Type 2 diabetes: (1) Sulfonylureas (e.g., glyburide [Micronase], glipizide [Glucotrol], and glimepiride [Amaryl]). Insulin is made in your pancreas, the gland that lies at the back of your belly. These drugs force the pancreas to make more insulin. (2) Biguanides (e.g., metformin [Glucophage]). These drugs limit the amount of sugar that is made by your liver. (3) a-Glucosidase inhibitors (e.g., acarbose [Precose] and miglitol [Glyset]). These drugs decrease the amount of sugar absorbed through your intestines. And (4) Thiazolidinediones (e.g., rosiglitazone [Avandia] and pioglitazone [Actos]). These drugs induce your muscles to use even more sugar than they normally do. As you can see, all these drugs aim to lower your sugar levels, by the variety of means described.

The first step in a newly diagnosed diabetic patient is usually weight reduction and the institution of an exercise program. Good control of diabetes, by whatever means necessary, will generally help in delaying or preventing coronary artery disease and other manifestations of arteriosclerosis. The development of diabetes mellitus does not necessarily mean that coronary artery disease is inevitable.

I smoke three packs of cigarettes a week. Does this increase my risk of developing coronary heart disease? How does smoking hurt my heart?

Cigarette smoking has been shown to be a very potent risk factor in causing premature coronary artery disease. The Framingham Heart Study places cigarette smoking among the three most serious risk factors, the other two being hypercholesterolemia (high cholesterol) and hypertension (high blood pressure). An individual who smokes three packs of cigarettes a week doubles the risk of developing premature coronary artery problems. The mechanism by which this occurs is not entirely known, but it is likely that some component of cigarette smoke is injurious to the lining of the coronary arteries and causes breakdown in the integrity of that layer. Once that occurs, then cholesterol, fat, and other atherosclerotic material can enter the wall of the artery, initiating the buildup of plaque or inducing narrowing. In addition to your heart, you are seriously damaging your lungs.

What is the French paradox?

It is somewhat of a mystery that the French have one of the lowest mortality rates from coronary artery disease. This is so in spite of the fact that the French consume large amounts of rich food laden with animal fat. The rate of coronary artery disease in France is comparable to that of European Mediterranean countries where the intake of saturated fat is lower. This is the French paradox. There are a number of theories as to why this paradox is so. Some say that the French also eat many fruits and vegetables, which counterbalances their meat intake. The most popular theory, however, is that the French consume a fair amount of alcohol, particularly in the form of wine, on a regular basis. A number of studies throughout the world have shown that moderate consumption of alcohol is associated with lower coronary artery disease rates. The reasons behind this finding may be related to the fact that moderate consumption of alcohol will lower LDL cholesterol, raise HDL cholesterol, and counteract the tendency of blood to clot. Red wine, in particular, decreases stickiness of platelets, part of the mechanism that leads to heart attack. However, it must be recognized that alcohol consumption may be habituating in certain individuals (alcoholism) and in itself it may lead to a variety of health, societal, and interpersonal problems.

Chapter
9
TREATMENT: MEDICATIONS, THERAPIES, AND PROCEDURES

MEDICATIONS

I have a diseased heart valve. Why does my cardiologist want me to take antibiotics? What do bacteria have to do with a heart valve?

I f you have a diseased heart valve—perhaps detected because of the presence of a heart murmur or found on an echocardiogram—that means that the inner lining of your heart is not as smooth as it should be and that flow patterns within the heart are turbulent, rather than laminar (smooth). These conditions—irregular surfaces and turbulent flow patterns—create an environment conducive to growth of bacteria.

Your doctor will, appropriately, insist that you take antibiotics if you should develop an infection (such as a boil or abscess), if you undergo dental work, or if you need intestinal or certain other kinds of surgery. Under such circumstances, bacteria can be liberated into your bloodstream and lodge in the abnormal valve(s), causing a serious internal infection of the heart. This can be prevented entirely by taking antibiotics promptly in case of infection *before* dental or surgical procedures.

What kinds of drugs are used to treat heart disease?

The accompanying figure shows some important classes of drugs that are often used to treat patients with heart disease. Many of these drugs are discussed more fully in pertinent sections of this book. Here we will look at the major classes of drugs based on the organ on which they exert their effects.

**Classes of Drugs Used
to Treat Heart Disease**

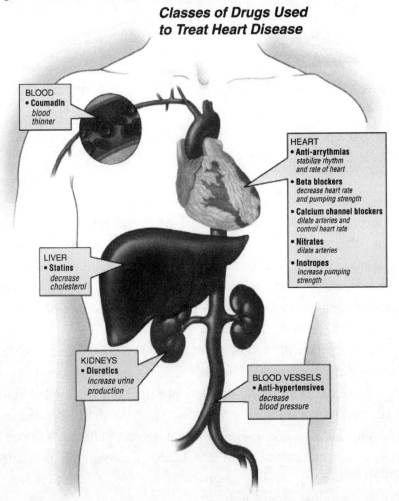

Figure 9.1. Classes of drugs used to treat heart disease (shown by target organ).

The blood. Blood thinners are often used to prevent clots from forming in different locations in your heart and your body. Antiplatelet drugs like aspirin or Plavix may be used to prevent clots from forming in your coronary arteries that could cause a heart attack (see figure 9.2). Such drugs also go under the names ticlopidine and clopidogrel. These same drugs may be used to keep an angioplasty site or a stent from closing. Coumadin is a powerful blood thinner used to prevent clots from forming on artificial heart valves or in the cardiac chambers in patients with atrial fibrillation.

The liver. Statins are powerful drugs that act on your liver to decrease the amount of cholesterol manufactured and liberated into your bloodstream.

The blood vessels. A whole class of drugs dilate your blood vessels, thus dropping the pressure that develops when the heart beats and ejects blood forcefully into your circulation. These drugs drop your blood pressure and are, accordingly, used to treat hypertension, or high blood pressure.

The kidneys. A class of drugs known as diuretics are used to promote formation and excretion of urine by your kidneys. These drugs are used to treat states of excess fluid retention, especially congestive heart failure. These drugs are also useful in combating hypertension. Lasix is among the best-known drugs in this class.

The heart itself. Antiarrhythmic drugs combat abnormal heart rhythms. Beta-blockers decrease the strength of cardiac contraction and are used for hypertension or angina. Calcium channel blockers dilate your arteries; they can be prescribed for both hypertension and angina, where they are used to dilate your coronary arteries. Nitrates are prescribed to dilate your coronary arteries (and sometimes other arteries as well). The well-known nitroglycerine tablets fall into this category. Inotropic agents are used to increase the strength of your heart's contraction, especially in cardiogenic shock or after major cardiac surgery.

You can locate more information on many of these drugs in the sections of this book that cover the specific cardiac diseases for which the drugs are used.

What is Coumadin?

Coumadin (also called Warfarin) is a blood thinner used for patients with mechanical heart valves (as well as for multiple other situations in medicine where clots need to be prevented). It is a pill taken once a day. It takes several days to build up to an effective level and, conversely, several days to wear off. It works by decreasing the ability of the liver to make the proteins that form blood clots, the so-called clotting factors.

Coumadin is monitored by a simple blood test called the INR or international normalized ratio. This test was developed specifically to promote uniformity of results throughout our country and the world, which can be very helpful to travelers. If your job or vacation takes you to France or Brazil or China or Australia, the INR will have the exact same meaning there as it does in your home state. And the INR is a very basic test that can be done in absolutely every clinical medical laboratory in the world. It is not an esoteric assay that requires a sophisticated, advanced medical environment.

The INR compares how quickly your blood clots relative to how quickly the blood of a patient who is not on Coumadin clots. The number shows quantitatively how many times longer your blood takes to clot. If your INR is 2, your blood takes twice as long as that of someone who is not on Coumadin; if your INR is 3, your blood takes three times as long. For mechanical valves in the aortic position, we usually like to run your INR at about 1.8 to 2.2. For mechanical valves in the mitral position, we like to run your INR at about 2.5 to 3.5. These are approximate ranges. Your surgeon, cardiologist, internist, or primary care practitioner may have his or her own ranges and preferences.

When you are first started on Coumadin in the hospital, you will have your INR checked daily. When you go home, you will probably have your INR checked two or three times a week. Thereafter, you will probably be checked on a weekly schedule. Eventually, you should be able to graduate to checking your INR only once every three months, especially if your diet and other medications are steady. Coumadin effectiveness is markedly influenced by many other medications. Some medications increase the potency of a given dose of Coumadin, and others decrease the potency. Any time that a medication is stopped or added, your Coumadin dosage will probably be monitored closely and adjusted. It is quite common for antibiotics to be started or discontinued early after your operation, and this can have a marked effect on your Coumadin regulation.

If you have underlying liver disease, especially from heavy drinking, you may be very sensitive to Coumadin.

Coumadin is a powerful pill in that it purposely decreases the speed and ease with which blood forms clots. As you might anticipate, Coumadin can exacerbate bleeding from internal problems or injuries. If you have a history of bleeding stomach ulcers, Coumadin may be especially dangerous for you. Likewise, if you have had bleeding from the urinary tract or the female tract, you may be vulnerable to complications from Coumadin. Also, if you have an aneurysm or other vascular problem in the brain, Coumadin may be very dangerous for you.

Certain activities are dangerous for patients on Coumadin. You should avoid contact sports (tackle football, wrestling) and sports in which falls are common (snow skiing, water skiing, horseback riding). If you were to fall and sustain bone fractures or internal injuries, you would bleed more than a patient not taking Coumadin.

You should pursue essentially all other activities vigorously and lead a very active life. Aerobic activities are not only permitted but encouraged. You will find that Coumadin will have a minimal impact on your lifestyle. Millions of patients in our country take this drug.

Pregnant women must not take Coumadin. Coumadin causes birth defects in the developing fetus. There are other options besides Coumadin, which your doctors can discuss with you. If you think you may be pregnant when Coumadin is prescribed for you, let your doctor know immediately. If you think you may become or may have become pregnant while taking Coumadin, again, notify your doctor immediately.

If any type of surgery is planned for you, you must let your doctor or dentist know that you are taking Coumadin, otherwise you could bleed excessively. There are means to take your Coumadin into account and render your upcoming operation safe, while still protecting your heart and heart valve. Your doctors can make these arrangements in advance, as long as you are certain to make them aware of your Coumadin treatment.

Who will adjust my Coumadin dosage?

Usually your internist or cardiologist will adjust your Coumadin dosage. In many offices, there is often a nurse who is a Coumadin specialist. She will review your Coumadin history and prior and current INR levels and prescribe any appropriate dose modifications, in consultation with your doctor. We suggest that you call the office managing your Coumadin and get an updated recommendation every time you have your INR checked.

In time, you will get to know your body and its response to Coumadin very well. The adjustment of dosage is a trial and error process. The dose is increased or decreased, and the subsequent changes in INR tested later. It is important to remember that effects of a dose change will not be fully manifested for at least several days after the alteration is made, due to the lag time for changes in your liver's metabolism.

There are devices available that permit patients to check their own INR from a pinprick performed at home (in the way that diabetics check their blood sugar).[1] In some trial programs, patients have adjusted their own Coumadin doses (again, like diabetics with their insulin). The consistency and accuracy of dose adjustment in trial programs have been fine, in some cases even better than with traditional doctor-based adjustments. These home INR testing systems are currently expensive, and have not been welcomed by the insurance industry. We anticipate, however, that within several years, many, if not most, patients will be testing their own INRs at home.

Can I drink if I am on Coumadin?

As everyone knows, drinking alcohol can adversely affect liver function. For a patient on Coumadin, the potential for adverse effects is very real. However, if your habit is to have a drink with your meals regularly, even daily, your Coumadin dosage can take this into account. Any changes in your regular routine, especially binges of heavy alcohol consumption, can be very dangerous to you. Such issues should be communicated frankly with your doctors.

What if I forget to take my Coumadin?

If you forget a daily dose or two, likely nothing will happen. We do not encourage this, of course. It is best if you take your Coumadin at a regular time each day. Most patients take their Coumadin after dinner. You can ask your family members to be sure to remind you. One or two missed doses will likely not have much impact. Were you to miss multiple doses, however, you would render yourself very vulnerable to clotting events.

How about aspirin; can I take aspirin if I am on Coumadin?

As you may be aware, aspirin and aspirin-containing medications, including over the counter preparations, can affect your blood clotting. Unlike Coumadin, which works on the manufacture of clotting proteins by your liver, aspirin directly impedes the function of the platelets in your blood. The platelets are the small cells that normally circulate in your blood and "plug" bleeding sites in your blood vessels. The platelets also help to induce and propagate clots by serving as points of attachment for the clotting proteins in the blood. See the schematic diagram of the clotting mechanism later in this chapter (fig. 9.2).

If you are on Coumadin and take aspirin as well, there is the potential for adverse additive impact on your blood clotting from the two mechanisms in which Coumadin and aspirin act. That is, you may impair both the clotting proteins and the platelets. This can make you vulnerable to bleeding. You should avoid aspirin and aspirin-containing medications if you take Coumadin. If you believe that you must take aspirin for some reason, you should contact your doctors first.

There are many other drugs that affect the platelets in the same way as aspirin. Many of these drugs fall in the category of nonsteroidal anti-inflammatory medications, that is, drugs, not steroids, which are used to decrease irritative reactions within the body. Arthritis is one example of an irritative process in the body that may be treated with such agents. These anti-inflammatory agents may be known as Cox-1 and Cox-2 inhibitors. Examples of names of these drugs include ibuprofen, Voltaren (diclofenac), and Vioxx (refocoxib). You should not start one of these medications without consulting your doctors first.

The Coumadin booklet says I can't ever have broccoli again. I love broccoli; what gives?

Broccoli and other green vegetables contain large amounts of vitamin K. This common vitamin is the substrate from which your liver makes the clotting proteins. Binging, or consuming an extraordinary volume of such vegetables, could overwhelm the ability of Coumadin to regulate your INR. Your Coumadin manuals will emphasize this possibility.

However, your authors have never, in decades of clinical practice, actually encountered an instance in which dietary intake of vegetables was a problem. Generally, you should plan to eat as you desire; your diet will automatically be accommodated in your INR testing and your Coumadin dosing. If you have an exceptionally large intake of green vegetables on a regular basis, discuss this with your doctors.

HYPERTENSION

What medications are available to treat high blood pressure?

There are a host of medications that have been developed over the past few decades to treat patients who have high blood pressure. These medications are of many different varieties:

1) Diuretics, for example, hydrochlorothiazide, furosemide
2) Beta-blockers, for example, propranolol, metoprolol, atenolol, nadolol
3) Calcium channel blockers, for example, nifedipine, verapamil, diltiazem
4) ACE (angiotensin converting enzyme) inhibitors, for example, captopril, enalapril, lisinopril, Monopril, fosinopril
5) ARB (angiotensin receptor blockers), for example, candesartan, irbesartan, losartan, valsartan, telmisartan

The above listing, though not exhaustive, does include the major classes of pharmaceutical drugs available to treat patients with hypertension. Side effects of these drugs vary, and a patient may have a reaction to a given agent but have no problems with another. For that reason, it is often necessary to try a variety of drugs before efficacy without side effects is achieved.

Table 9.1. Classes of Drugs.

Class of Drugs	How They Work	Examples	Side Effects
Diuretics	Drive out fluid through increased urine production	Hydrochlorthiazide (Hydrodiuril) Furosemide (Lasix)	Dizziness Fainting Kidney dysfunction Low potassium
Beta-blockers	Decrease force of heart contraction	Propranolol (Inderal) Nadolol (Corgard) Metoprolol (Lopressor)	Dizziness Tiredness Sexual dysfunction

		Atenolol (Tenormin) Carvedilol (Coreg)	
Calcium channel blockers	Decrease force of cardiac contraction (except nifedipine). Dilate arteries	Nifedipine (Adalat) Verapamil (Calan) (Isoptin) Diltiazem (Cardizem)	Dizziness Swelling
ACE-inhibitors (angiotensin converting enzyme inhibitors)	Dilate arteries	Captopril (Capoten) Enalapril (Vasotec) Lisinopril (Prinivil) (Zestril) Fosinopril (Monopril)	Dizziness Kidney dysfunction
ARBs (angio-tensin receptor blockers)	Dilate arteries	Candesartan (Atacand) Irbesartan (Avapro) Losartan (Cozaar) Valsartan (Diovan) Telmisartan (Micardis)	Dizziness Kidney dysfunction

HIGH CHOLESTEROL

What medications are available to treat my high cholesterol?

If careful diet and regular exercise are not enough to keep your cholesterol in line, multiple medications are available that can help to bring down your levels.

For decades physicians have sought medications to lower cholesterol levels. Early attempts were in general not successful. Recognizing that women tended to have a lower incidence of coronary disease than did men, some researchers performed an early trial of giving men with severe coronary disease female estrogen hormones.[2] This proved to be unsuccessful for many reasons.

The next advance was the development of a class of drugs called bile acid sequestrants, such as cholestyramine. They acted by binding cholesterol in the gastrointestinal tract. Their side effects—constipation, bloating, flatulence, and abdominal pain—made them quite unpopular. Few but the most motivated patients could tolerate taking them for any period of time.

Another class of agents called the fibrates, such as gemfibrozil (Fenofibrate), were also utilized. The results of these drugs varied. Although cholesterol levels dropped modestly, the incidence of death did not necessarily decrease.[3]

The vitamin niacin has a modest effect on lowering both cholesterol and triglycerides, but large doses must be taken. This often results in a side effect of flushing, which makes this medication unacceptable. Niacin may also have undesirable effects upon the liver.

A bit over a decade ago, another class of agents, called statins, were developed. These drugs, which impair the liver's ability to manufacture cholesterol, have revolutionized the clinical field of cholesterol lowering. Lovastatin (Mevacor) was the first statin drug approved for use. Since then, fluvastatin (Lescol), atorvastatin (Lipitor), pravastatin (Pravachol), and simvastatin (Zocor) have all been introduced. These drugs have been shown to be beneficial both in arresting established coronary artery disease as well as in preventing the onset of coronary artery disease. In general, these medications are remarkably free of side effects and are tolerated well.

The most recently introduced statin, cerivastatin (Baycol), has just been removed from the market after a number of patients developed kidney failure due to muscle breakdown.[4] Most of these patients had combined cerivastatin with a fibrate, a combination that is always to be avoided.

I have heard that the statin drugs are beneficial in some other way besides decreasing my cholesterol. Can you explain that to me?

You are correct. Evidence is accumulating that the statin drugs have an unexpected, unanticipated, but powerful additional beneficial effect. Many drug discoveries occur by chance, and this is one of them.

Specifically, it appears that the statins, by some unknown mechanism, stabilize arteriosclerotic plaques. By this we mean that the statins seem to prevent plaques from rupturing and leading to clotting in the artery and to heart attack. Remember that we feel that many heart attacks are triggered by rupture of the cap over a plaque. Statins seem to prevent this. Statins are important for this reason as well as for their lowering of cholesterol. Also, the statins seem to inhibit the inflammation, or irritation, in and around arteriosclerotic plaques, which is a very beneficial effect.

ARTERIOSCLEROSIS AND CORONARY HEART DISEASE

Can any medications make my coronary artery blockages go away?

The simple answer to this question is no. If you saw the nature of the blockages that we encounter every day in the operating room, you would understand this answer. The arteriosclerosis eventually becomes calcified, or filled with calcium. Calcium is the building block of bone, and the arteriosclerotic lesions in coronary arteries become as hard as bone. We often comment to medical students that the arteries we are going to have them feel during a bypass operation will seem to them like nonbiologic structures. Biologic structures are soft and pliable, whereas severely affected coronary arteries feel like steel brake lines from a car. A disease that has progressed to calcification will not go away with any nonsurgical treatment.

The lipid-lowering statin agents can, however, stabilize arteriosclerotic lesions so that they do not progress further. In very few instances, soft lesions can improve somewhat on vigorous medical therapy, but the levels of improvement are usually slight.

A word should be said about claims to reverse arteriosclerosis with unconventional therapies, such as the widely touted chelation therapy. Simply put, there is no widely accepted scientific data supporting regression of coronary artery lesions on chelation therapy. While it is important for physicians in general to have open minds toward emerging or alternative therapies, despite decades of promotion of chelation therapy, accepted scientific proof of its utility is still lacking.

How will the doctor treat my angina?

There are several mainstays of angina treatment. Nitroglycerine tablets dissolved under the tongue are taken as needed to treat an episode of angina as it is developing. A long-acting nitroglycerine preparation, taken orally as a tablet or in the form of a transdermal patch, is given to help prevent future anginal episodes. A class of agents called beta-blockers are a mainstay in the treatment of angina because of a variety of beneficial mechanisms, all of which cut down on the workload of the heart and decrease the heart muscle's oxygen needs. Calcium channel blockers dilate the coronary arteries, and some of these agents also decrease the workload of the heart.

If medication is not effective in alleviating angina and improving the quality of life, a balloon angioplasty (PTCA) or coronary artery bypass grafting (CABG) may be appropriate interventions.

How does nitroglycerine work?

Nitroglycerine is really a miracle drug. Nitroglycerine has even forged a role for itself in books, television, and movies. The image of a middle-aged character clutching his chest and popping a nitro tablet under his tongue is familiar to all.

Nitroglycerine is an extremely effective medication, able to relieve all but the most severe angina attacks.

How does nitroglycerine relieve angina? This is accomplished through two mechanisms.

First, nitroglycerine dilates the coronary arteries, the arteries that supply blood to the heart. By dilating the coronary arteries, nitroglycerine allows more blood to flow to your oxygen-starved heart muscle. Of course, nitroglycerine, powerful as it is, cannot dilate severe blockages caused by arteriosclerosis, which may even be rock-hard from calcium deposition. But nitroglycerine will dilate all segments that are amenable, and it usually increases dramatically the amount of blood flow to your heart.

Second, nitroglycerine dilates the large veins in your body, especially those in your legs. This pools or sequesters blood out of the main circulatory stream of your body. This is good for the angina patient because, by decreasing the venous blood returning to the heart that needs to be pumped forward, nitroglycerine decreases the workload on your heart. With less work to do, your troubled heart requires less blood and less oxygen. Thus, the amount of blood flow available through the coronary arteries becomes relatively more sufficient.

Thus, the miracle drug nitroglycerine works in two supplementary ways: it increases the nourishing blood available to your heart muscle and decreases the amount of blood required by your heart. Nitroglycerine increases supply and decreases demand for blood and oxygen by your heart. This is all greatly beneficial and explains why nitroglycerine is so effective at relieving chest pain.

Another part of the miracle of this drug, which has been used for over a hundred years, is that it is absorbed almost immediately into your bloodstream when you place the tablet under your tongue. The so-called mucous membranes under your tongue are rich in blood vessels, which absorb the nitroglycerine as it dissolves and carry it into your bloodstream. This is why nitroglycerine works so rapidly. You can expect your angina attack to be relieved within minutes.

So important is nitroglycerine that it is available not only in the form of the well-known sublingual tablets but also as ordinary pills to be swallowed in the usual fashion for sustained effect. In this latter form, nitroglycerine may be known as Isordil or Imdur. Also, nitroglycerine is available as sustained-release patches that are placed on the skin.

I am taking more and more nitroglycerine. I use these pills almost like candy. Is that OK?

No, that is definitely not OK. Angina attacks are serious business. Although some patients have the attacks with some regularity, especially with severe exertion, if the pattern—the frequency and severity and duration—is increasing, that constitutes what we call *unstable angina*. Unstable angina often indicates that a heart attack is looming. If you are using nitro more frequently, or taking more nitro pills to control specific angina attacks, you must let your doctor know promptly. In fact, if one or two nitro pills do not relieve a specific episode of pain, a heart attack may be starting. You need to let your doctor know right away. If you cannot reach your doctor, you should go immediately to the nearest emergency room.

Why is aspirin so important?

Aspirin, although a very old and cheap product, is really a wonder drug. In the case of patients with heart disease, aspirin is useful because of its "antithrombotic," or clot-preventing, properties.

Why is this significant? Well, we feel that most heart attacks begin when the inner lining—or endothelium—of the coronary artery is injured, exposing the underlying layers. The underlying layers, not being covered by the smooth cells lining the endothelium, are quite "thrombogenic," or clot inducing. The heart attack occurs when a clot forms on those clot-inducing exposed cells, resulting eventually in a sudden blockage of the artery. Aspirin can stop this entire clotting process from occurring. It does this by disabling a crucial enzyme that makes platelets clump together to form blood clots. Aspirin will cut the chance of a second heart attack, in those who have suffered a first, by 25 percent. We believe that aspirin is also effective in preventing first heart attacks, but this has not been proven as conclusively at this time.

Aspirin may have yet another important role. As mentioned in the section above on risk factors for coronary artery disease, there is increasing suspicion that *inflammation*, the medical term for irritation, of the arteries plays a significant role in causing subsequent arteriosclerosis. Aspirin, we know, is a powerful anti-inflammatory agent. This is why so many people use aspirin to treat arthritis, an inflammation of the joints. So, it is quite possible that the anti-inflammatory as well as the antithrombotic properties of aspirin are vital to the heart.

Most doctors recommend that those with known coronary artery disease and those at significant risk of developing coronary artery disease (because of family history or a high cholesterol level, for example) take an aspirin daily. This can be either a baby aspirin (75 milligrams) or an adult aspirin (325 milligrams).

As most patients are aware, aspirin may irritate the stomach lining and even cause bleeding from the stomach or intestines. Those with a history of ulcers or stomach trouble should be cautious in using aspirin, even for the benefit of the heart. Certainly, if you note gastric distress or heartburn after starting a daily aspirin regimen, you should stop. For all patients, it is best to ask your doctor if he approves of your taking an aspirin each day specifically for its cardiac-protective benefits.

A very recent study shows that patients taking the anti-inflammatory agent ibuprofen in addition to aspirin may lose the cardio-protective effects of the aspirin.[5] This combination of medications should probably be avoided.

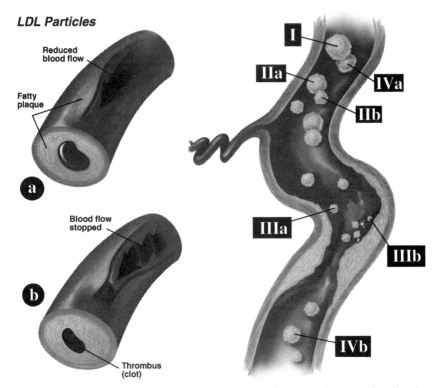

Figure 9.2. The process of clot development at the site of an arteriosclerotic lesion, leading from partial restriction to complete cessation of blood flow and a heart attack. Note how the lipid particles (of various subtypes) accumulate along the sides of the coronary artery. Flow eventually becomes so slow that the blood clots, which leads to a heart attack. Aspirin, while it cannot prevent the accumulation of lipid deposits, can prevent the final formation of a clot. In discouraging this clotting process, aspirin can actually prevent a heart attack from occurring.

Recently Vioxx was taken off the market by its manufacturer. It was the best medicine I ever tried for relief of pain in my knees due to osteoarthritis. Is it really dangerous?

Vioxx belongs to a class of pain relief medications called Cox-2 inhibitors. Whereas Cox-2 inhibitors cut down on the pain associated with an inflammatory site, they also increase the ability of blood to clot. Studies have suggested that the incidence of heart attack and stroke are increased in individuals taking Vioxx. The manufacturer therefore took this drug off the market in September 2005.[6] Two other Cox-2 inhibitors, Bextra and Celebrex, are still available, but there is some concern that they, too, may increase the incidence of heart attack and stroke. The final word on all three drugs is still not in.

What is a balloon angioplasty?

In 1979 a Swiss physician described a small number of patients who had undergone a balloon angioplasty. This is a procedure—which continues today—wherein a catheter with an attached balloon is placed inside a coronary artery at the site of a narrowing or plaque. The balloon is then inflated, causing the plaque to transfigure and thereby open up the coronary artery channel by which blood nourishes the heart muscle. The frequency of the procedure has grown in the United States from one thousand per year when first introduced to over four hundred thousand per year currently. Dramatic worldwide growth in this procedure has been realized as well.

Are there other techniques that can open a coronary artery?

The balloon angioplasty has remained the cornerstone of this type of technique. However, over the past eight years, a refinement of the method has evolved. The majority of patients undergoing balloon angioplasty currently receive a stent. A stent is a device that is deployed as the balloon is inflated. The stent is similar to a mesh or to a piece of an erector set. As the balloon is inflated, the mesh becomes embedded in the wall of the coronary artery, helping to keep the lumen open and safe from collapsing.

Laser therapy has virtually been abandoned, as the long-term results most often led to scarring of the vessel. But a catheter that has a shaving knife attached is sometimes utilized. This technique is called direct atherectomy. Finally, a Rotablator, similar to a high-speed dentist's drill, has been used for a small number of patients. Anatomic details of a specific blockage in a specific patient may suggest that one of these alternative technical devices be applied. However, the balloon angioplasty with stenting remains the most commonly used nonsurgical intervention.

Angioplasty

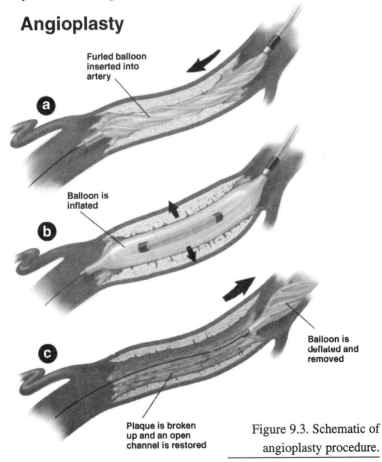

Furled balloon inserted into artery

a

Balloon is inflated

b

Balloon is deflated and removed

c

Plaque is broken up and an open channel is restored

Figure 9.3. Schematic of angioplasty procedure.

What about these drug-coated stents that I have been hearing about? What does the drug coating do?

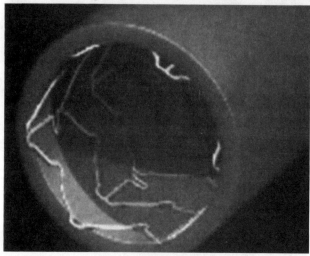

Figure 9.4. Schematic of coronary artery stent, courtesy of Guidant Corporation. Note how the fine metal mesh of the stent supports and "girds" the wall of the vessel, preventing it from collapsing or narrowing.

A stent by itself is effective in the short term, but the stented site often narrows in the long term. Medical science was looking for a method to prevent that long-term narrowing, known technically as *late restenosis*. The answer seems to have been found in the drug-eluting stents.

These stents are coated with a drug that prevents a scar from forming as a reaction of the body to the foreign metal of the stent. Actually, the drug with which the stent is coated comes from the family of medications used to prevent the body from rejecting transplanted organs. The drug coating gradually "leaches" out from the stent, providing a durable prevention of local scarring.

Drug-eluting stents have markedly reduced the incidence of in-

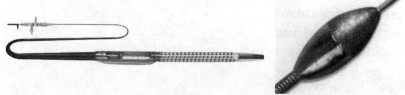

Figures 9.5 left and 9.5 right. Schematic of atherectomy and Rotablator devices, courtesy of Guidant Corporation. These devices are like miniature "drills" or "reamers," which clear a path through a blocked artery.

stent restenosis—repeat narrowing within the stented area—to about the single-digit percentage range. This has been a major advance in angioplasty techniques.

Some very recent information, however, may indicate a kink in the armor, so to speak—almost as if the benefit of drug-eluting stents was too good to be true. In the last several years, we have found that some patients with drug-eluting stents die suddenly from abrupt heart attacks. We have found that these deaths are related to sudden thrombosis (clotting) of the stented artery. It appears that this occurs mainly in patients who stop taking the antiplatelet drugs prescribed after drug-eluting stent placement. Specifically, a powerful drug called Plavix, which makes the platelets nonsticky, preventing clotting, is an essential adjunct after placement of a drug-eluting stent. This drug may be maintained long-term. When it is stopped abruptly, then clotting and heart attack can occur.[7]

It appears that the rate of sudden closure of the drug-eluting stent site accounts for about a 2 percent per year death rate. This is a very large number. In fact, you should discuss with your heart doctor whether coronary artery bypass may be a preferable alternative to placement of a drug-eluting stent in your particular case. This is a topic of debate between cardiologists, who perform stenting, and cardiac surgeons, who perform the bypass procedure. You will likely want to speak with both to get a fuller picture.

How can I tell if an angioplasty would suffice, or if I need bypass surgery?

Angioplasty is ideally performed on a symptomatic patient who has narrowing in one or two coronary arteries. There are many patients, however, who have more diffuse narrowing involving three or more coronary arteries. Such patients usually benefit from having coronary artery bypass surgery. The restenosis rate in each artery undergoing balloon angioplasty may approach 10 to 15 percent. Therefore, if three arteries undergo angioplasty, the likelihood of stenosis in one of them becomes considerable. In addition, the ideal candidate for angioplasty is the patient who has narrowing in the beginning part of the artery. If the narrowings are farther downstream, then surgery becomes a more attractive option. Also, there is some evidence that diabetics do not fare as well after angioplasty. So for many diabetics, surgery is preferred. Finally, if the left main coronary artery has a significant stenosis, then surgery is the treatment of choice.

Also, if angioplasty has been performed once or more already, and the blockage has returned, surgery is often preferred.

The choice between angioplasty and surgery is at times a judgment call. The patient may well have preferences, and his opinion is a major factor in our choice of therapies. Some of the factors patient and doctor may put to bear on the decision are listed in the accompanying table.

Table 9.2. Factors Bearing on Decision Making:
Angioplasty versus Surgery.

	Favor Angioplasty	**Favor Surgery**
No. of diseased vessels	One or two	Three
No. of blockages per vessel	One	Multiple
Focal vs. diffuse disease	Focal	Diffuse
Partial vs. total blockage	Partial	Total
Left main lesion	Not appropriate	Necessary
Diabetes	Less favorable	Preferred
Prior angioplasty(ies)	Less enthusiasm	Preferred

How long will the results of the angioplasty last?

The results of angioplasty have improved steadily over the years, especially with the addition of stents to support the angioplasty site. Very preliminary results from Europe indicate that new antibiotic-impregnated stents may achieve even further improvement in angioplasty results. Nonetheless, coronary artery bypass surgery remains the gold standard for long-term effectiveness. Nearly all mammary-based bypasses remain patent (functioning) for the remainder of the patient's life. Vein bypasses usually function for six to ten years or longer. Generally, angioplasty results are measured on a shorter timescale of months to years. Also, the more arteries that require an angioplasty, the greater the likelihood that at least one will recur.

For an individual patient, the decision often boils down to a selection between the more reliable and durable bypass operation versus the less invasive angioplasty procedure.

Also, it comes as no surprise that the two classes of heart specialists, cardiologists and surgeons, both prefer their own special procedures. Thus, cardiologists often favor angioplasty and surgeons often favor surgery. In patients with multiple blockages in multiple vessels, usually both specialists settle on a recommendation for surgery.

I've been told that doctors are "procedure happy." Should I be concerned that an unnecessary procedure may be done on me?

This is not a silly question. Doctors, hospitals, and clinics are under tremendous pressure to do procedures, as procedures determine reimbursement from insurers and the government. The number of procedures can impact salaries or even the fiscal viability of a program or a hospital. The impact of these pressures can be enormous.

These forces notwithstanding, your authors can attest that unnecessary procedures are not at all common in the multiple academic settings in which we have worked. The vast majority of heart specialists are highly principled and have the patient's future safety and cardiac health as their sole goals. Also, there are safeguards in terms of standards set by the American College of Cardiology.

In terms of surgery for your heart, there is a built-in safeguard in the very fact that you usually do not get referred to a surgeon until an independent cardiologist has determined that you need a cardiac operation. Thus, there are checks and balances at work. The doctor who makes the referral is not the one who does the operation. Incentive issues are obviated in this way.

In the case of angioplasty, often the same doctor who performs the diagnostic catheterization is the one who performs the angioplasty procedure. Some experts are concerned about this lack of independent confirmation of the necessity for the procedure.

In fact, the American Heart Association has insisted on focused sessions on this particular concern. The American Heart Association has, tongue-in-cheek, dubbed this bias toward the performance of angioplasty the very moment that the cardiologist demonstrates a blockage as "the oculo-stenotic"reflex." This refers to a reflex-type phenomenon not in you, the patient, but in your *doctor*! This term, humorously intended in part, is meant to signify that the moment an invasive cardiologist sees a blockage, he has an almost irresistible impulse to stretch it with an angioplasty balloon. First, stretching these blockages represents his specialized expertise; he has trained years and years to develop the skills and knowledge to perform this advanced therapy. Second, he may have financial gain from performing the angioplasty. Furthermore, the decision to perform angioplasty is often made instantly on the spot, as the patient is already in the catheterization laboratory and the catheters are already in place.

What we suggest is the following. Be sure to discuss the issue of angioplasty with your cardiologist before you enter the laboratory for your diagnostic catheterization. Request that options be discussed with you (if you are alert enough) or with your family if blockages amenable to angioplasty should be discovered. Medical management may be an alternative to angioplasty in some cases. Also, you should feel free to request a second opinion. No proper physician should ever be dismayed at your request for another learned opinion. It is your health and your life that are at stake. Decisions are often matters of judgment. Most excellent cardiac specialists welcome second opinions, provided that the clinical circumstances are stable enough to permit the time necessary to solicit and obtain a second consultation.

Above all, be comfortable with your selection of a cardiac specialist. Often your general practitioner, your internist, or friends or family can make a referral to a specialist whom they have come to know and trust. And, remember, most cardiologists, as in every field, are aboveboard and ethical.

HEART FAILURE

How will the doctor treat my congestive heart failure?

In congestive heart failure, the heart is deficient in its pumping strength, so that blood becomes backed up behind the pumping chambers. When it is the left ventricle that is at fault, we call the situation *left heart failure*. In this circumstance, blood backs up in the lungs, causing wet lungs and shortness of breath. If the situation is extremely severe, with profound shortness of breath, it is called *pulmonary edema.*

If the right ventricle is pumping insufficiently, blood backs up

Case 1. Playing the Odds.

Mr. Fulton was an insurance reinsurer—buying and selling large bulks of insurance policies between underwriters. He had a mind for statistics, and he put his mind to work with the information that the doctors at the Heart Failure Clinic were providing. He would be gone in three months unless he took the plunge—but a huge plunge it was—to go for the artificial heart.

His life had been remarkable. He had been to Vietnam. He had raced Formula 1 with the great Peter Revson. He had played some semipro hockey, and now coached a Little League team. But his greatest accomplishment, in his own mind, was getting his wonderful wife, Cathy, to marry him. He adored Cathy, and she him. They had produced accomplished children and a bevy of grandchildren.

But the last ten years had been hell. A large heart attack had weakened his heart dramatically. A defibrillator had been implanted. The heart had grown bigger and weaker each year. Big is good in many ways, but not so far as the heart is concerned. The heart only grows big as a last-ditch effort by nature to keep the blood flowing. If each heartbeat is weak, just a trace of a squeeze, a little more blood will be propelled by a larger heart. Medication after medication had been added to aid the failing heart. Taking the drugs accurately and on time had become a full-time endeavor.

And now he needed to be in the hospital all the time, getting powerful diuretics by vein, as well as a powerful tonic medication for the heart from a mechanical administration pump beside the bed.

Mr. Fulton played the statistics in his mind. Sure, there were risks from the artificial heart, and especially from the operation to place it. But without surgery, the numbers showed he would not live to see his youngest grandchild start kindergarten.

"Let's do it," he said. He had used the same words thirty-eight years earlier when he and Revson were preparing to race at Le Mans.

in the body, especially the legs and the belly. In the legs, the excess fluid is called *edema*. In the belly, it is called *ascites*.

Most often, although not always, right and left heart failure go hand-in-hand. The accompanying figure shows a patient with all the major symptoms of heart failure.

As you might imagine, diuretics, or water pills, are used in congestive heart failure to help the body excrete excess fluid. These are very effective drugs, which are the mainstay of treatment of congestive heart failure.

If you have heart failure, your doctor may also give you digitalis, also known as digoxin. This oral medication mildly increases the strength of your heart's contraction.

Your doctor may give you drugs that dilate your arteries, such as those used to treat hypertension. These drugs make it easier for your failing heart to propel blood forward.

It may seem paradoxical, but the beta-blockers, which decrease heart rate and strength of heart contraction, have in recent years been found to ameliorate heart failure symptoms. The mechanism of this improvement is not entirely clear. Nonetheless, it is likely that your doctor will place you on one of these drugs.

Ultimately, it is hoped that some mechanical problem is the cause of your heart failure, because these types of problems can be corrected by surgery. If your problem is caused by a narrowed or leaky heart valve, that can be corrected by an operation. If your heart failure is related to blocked coronary arteries, you can have a coronary bypass operation. Heart failure symptoms can be improved dramatically when they are amenable to a condition that can be addressed by an operation.

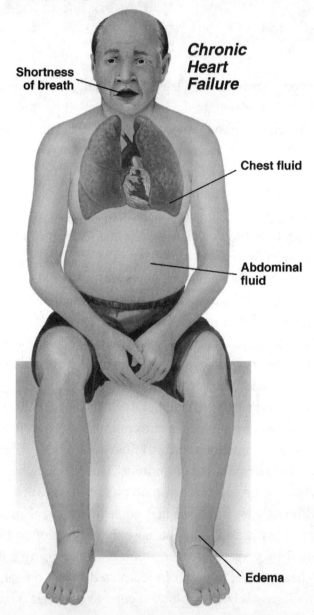

Figure 9.6. A patient with the typical features of chronic heart failure.

Why is potassium so important?

The diuretic pills (such as Lasix) that your doctor may prescribe to encourage your kidneys to excrete the excess fluid caused by heart failure may deplete your body's potassium. Urine is generally potassium-rich. The more urine you make, the more potassium you lose.

Now, potassium is a chemical element that is extremely vital to your heart. Potassium stabilizes the electrical function of your heart cells and the conducting, or electrical, system of your heart. When potassium is depleted, your heart becomes electrically irritable. The end result is arrhythmias of the heart. These arrhythmias may include ventricular tachycardia or ventricular fibrillation, which are life-threatening or even fatal. Thus, if you neglect to take your potassium, you are putting your heart and your very life in jeopardy. Simply put, neglect your potassium and you die.

Patients with prior history of arrhythmia, prior heart attack, poor pumping strength of the heart, or recent heart surgery are especially prone to serious arrhythmias from potassium depletion.

But my potassium pills taste so bad, I can't stand it.

There is no question that potassium is concentrated and caustic. Certain patients find it particularly unsavory. It can certainly irritate the stomach.

If you prefer, you can generally substitute certain potassium-rich foods for each tablet of potassium. A banana, an orange, or a cup of broth will all provide you with a generous amount of potassium. You can substitute one or two of the above for each potassium pill, but this must be done reliably and without fail, or you will be putting your life in jeopardy.

If you are taking diuretics, your doctor will probably monitor your potassium level periodically. Although there is some minor variation from laboratory to laboratory, we usually like to see your potassium from 4.0 to 5.0 milliequivalent per liter (abbreviated meq/L).

I'm not taking diuretics. Can potassium still help my heart?

No, you must not take potassium if you are not on diuretics. High potassium levels can be equally dangerous to your heart. If your potassium level is too high, your heart may actually stop. That is precisely how we stop your heart's function for the purpose of conducting open heart surgery; we deliberately raise the potassium level.

Your body regulates the potassium level very accurately, but you can overwhelm your body's ability to regulate by taking excess potassium. This powerful element, potassium, is not a vitamin. You should not under any circumstances take it without your doctor's prescription.

What is this new "miracle drug" that I have heard about for heart failure?

There is indeed a promising new type of drug for heart failure called nesiritide (Natrecor). This is unlike any traditional drugs previously used to treat heart failure, but it is certainly too early to call it a "miracle" treatment. In fact, the drug has just recently been approved for clinical use.

Natrecor is artificially produced to mimic a hormone naturally secreted by the heart muscle in response to heart failure. Natrecor lowers the backup of pressure in the lungs due to heart failure.

Natrecor is available only in intravenous form. Its use is confined to hospitalized patients with advanced and decompensated heart failure. It is not applicable to patients being treated at home for chronic, compensated heart failure. Stable, out-of-hospital patients still need to be treated conventionally, as outlined above.

If you should need to be admitted to the hospital for a severe acute episode of heart failure, you may well be treated with Natrecor for your immediate management.

Does everyone with heart failure need a transplant?

The answer to this question is an emphatic no. The vast majority of patients with heart failure can be effectively treated with medications (see above). Only those who are most severely affected become candidates for heart transplantation.

The decision to explore heart transplantation as an alternative is usually predicated on one of two factors: (1) If the patient's quality of life is severely affected, transplantation should be explored. (2) If tests indicate that the patient's survival will be severely curtailed, even with optimal medical monitoring and treatment, then transplantation becomes an option. We will explore each of these indications more fully.

The classification of the severity of heart failure is explained in chapter 2 in the section "How do you grade the severity of heart failure?" If the patient has shortness of breath with even mild or no exertion (placing him in New York Heart Association Class III or IV), then he usually cannot lead a satisfying, fulfilling live. If he cannot breathe comfortably, if he cannot walk around the house or outdoors for even short distances, if he is distressed even when sitting and watching TV or reading, or if he cannot sleep without being awakened by breathing distress, then life may not be worth living. Episodes of what we call *respiratory distress*, or difficulty breathing, are often terrifying to the patient, like repeated episodes of drowning. When such advanced states continue despite the best medications available, patients beg for something more to be done. That something more is heart transplantation. In the present day, mechanical heart replacement (with one of the multiple brands of artificial heart devices currently available) represents another alternative.

This classification also has direct implications in terms of the patient's survival outlook. Of all patients with only Class I heart failure, over 50 percent will be alive five years later. Of those patients developing Class IV heart failure, however, over 50 percent of them will lose their lives to heart disease during the first year. See the accompanying figure.

The patient with heart failure will have a number of tests aimed at assessing the likelihood that his heart disease will take his life in the near future. One such test is the evaluation of his ejection fraction (see above). This may be done with an echocardiogram or a nuclear exam (MUGA or ERNA scan). These tests are discussed above in the preceding chapter on tests. As you will recall from our earlier discussion, the normal ejection fraction is 55 percent to 65 percent. Patients with heart failure often have an ejection fraction below 30 percent. When the calculated values of ejection fraction fall to the 10 percent to 20 percent range, the heart has become very, very weak and may not hold up much longer.

Another test your doctor will order is an exercise test designed to measure your capacity to utilize oxygen. This is basically a test of how in shape you are. The results are usually measured in terms of the maximum number of ml/kg/min (milliliters per kilogram per minute) of oxygen that you can use while exercising. A normal patient, even above age sixty, can achieve more than 20 ml/kg/min of oxygen utilization. If your heart is pumping weakly, you will not be able to exercise to such levels. If the heart is very weak, patients may be able only to reach 10 to 15 ml/kg/min before shortness of breath or exhaustion forces them to stop exercising. We know that patients with exercise capacity as low as that range have a very poor outlook, with a high likelihood of death in the near future.

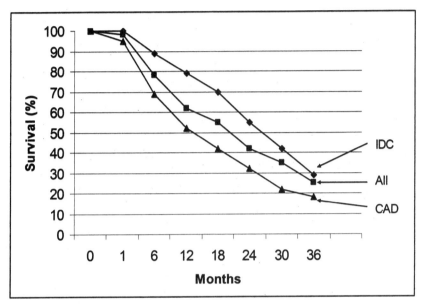

Figure 9.7. Poor prognosis for severe heart failure. Note the dismal survival curves for patients with heart failure. IDC stands for idiopathic dilated cardiomyopathy, or heart failure of uncertain cause. CAD stands for heart failure due to coronary artery disease. All represents all patients in both the IDC and CAD categories.[8]

Your doctor will also likely order a test to see if you are suffering from frequent bouts of arrhythmia, especially ventricular tachycardia. These abnormal heart rhythms are discussed above. As you will recall from the corresponding section of this book, the test called a "Holter monitor" actually records every heartbeat for a twenty-hour period. By analyzing the tape, your doctor will determine if you are having frequent or repeated episodes of the very dangerous ventricular tachycardia. If so, you are at risk for sudden cardiac death in the near future.

Most patients referred for heart transplantation can be expected to have only a 50 percent chance of surviving the next six months without a transplant operation.

The other factor that your doctor will consider in determining whether you should pursue transplantation is the direction in which your heart health is going. If you are feeling progressively more poorly, if your ejection fraction is falling, if your exercise capacity is deteriorating, and if you are showing more arrhythmias, then more than likely transplantation should be considered.

How could I have gotten heart failure so severe that I could need a heart transplant?

There are two common ways by which a patient can get heart failure and come to require heart transplantation. The first is through a heart attack or multiple heart attacks. Heart attack means necrosis, or death, of heart muscle through the blockage of one of the three arteries supplying blood to the heart. This, of course, results from arteriosclerosis, or hardening of the arteries. When this happens suddenly, a heart attack ensues, and a chunk of heart muscle is lost. The heart has a limited reserve of muscle, and a single very large attack, or multiple smaller attacks, can cause heart failure. This dangerous path accounts for about half of all heart failure cases.

The other half of cases are caused by viruses, of the same type as those that can give you a runny nose and a sore throat. These viruses can get hold of the heart muscle and not let go until it is nearly destroyed. Because the original viral event is usually not known or recognized, these cases of heart failure seem to arise out of the blue, often in otherwise healthy, young people without cardiac risk factors. For this reason, such cases are referred to as "idiopathic cardiomyopathy," which is Greek for weakness of the heart muscle due to unknown causes. In other words, although sometimes there is a smoking gun of high viral concentrations even years later, there is not a direct cause and effect relationship that we can see at the time that the heart failure occurs.

In general, heart failure from hardening of the arteries occurs in older patients, aged forty-five and above. But the viral infection can occur in young patients, even in children and teenagers.

These are the two major causes of heart failure. There are some additional cases due to neglected valvular disease, severe hypertension, congenital heart disease, and the like.

ARRHYTHMIA

You will recall the case of Mrs. Matthews, the ophthalmologist's mother who was intolerant of her atrial fibrillation. Through a combination of digoxin and blocking medications, one of the authors controlled her heart rate so that she became no longer distressed by, or even aware of, the irregular cardiac rhythm. The general approach to atrial fibrillation and other arrhythmias is described below.

How will the doctor treat my atrial fibrillation?

There are several goals in the treatment of atrial fibrillation. The first goal is to determine if the heart rhythm can be brought back to a normal sinus rhythm. You will remember from chapter 3 that "normal sinus rhythm" is the standard rhythm of the heart. Restoration of normal sinus rhythm is most readily accomplished by a procedure called an electrical cardioversion, the administration of a synchronized shock to convert the atrial fibrillation rhythm back to normal. If atrial fibrillation has been going for twenty-four hours or more, the cardioversion procedure may be preceded by a transesophageal echocardiogram to make certain that no blood clots have formed in the left atrium during the abnormal rhythm. Alternatively, the doctor may decide to anticoagulate the patient (that is, to give him blood thinners) for three to four weeks so that if any clots had formed they would dissolve. These maneuvers are performed because the highest risk of a clot dislodging from the heart and traveling to a vital organ occurs at the time of conversion from atrial fibrillation to a normal rhythm.

The reason for preferring sinus rhythm to atrial fibrillation is that the patient with atrial fibrillation has a four to five percent annual incidence of a clot forming and traveling from the heart. This is lessened by continuous anticoagulation, but patients on long-term anticoagulation do face an increased incidence of bleeding.

Not all cases of atrial fibrillation can be converted to normal sinus rhythm. For cases that persist, it then becomes imperative for the doctor to use medications to control the heart rate. This is necessary because, in atrial fibrillation, the heart rate can be very rapid. Rates of 100, 140, and even 180 beats per minute are seen. Your doctor will usually use digoxin, a powerful medication, to bring your heart rate down toward normal. Digoxin is unique in that it drops the rate of atrial fibrillation without decreasing the heart's strength of contraction. Digoxin by itself usually is not sufficient. Your doctor will usually add a beta-blocker and/or a calcium channel blocker in addition to digoxin. We usually aim to control the heart rate in atrial fibrillation to 100 beats or less per minute.

Atrial fibrillation tends to be a recurrent problem. It can at times be prevented from recurring by the use of antiarrhythmic drugs. If this is not the case, a procedure called "catheter ablation" may be undertaken. This procedure resembles a cardiac catheterization, but the catheter used is one that is able to produce radiofrequency energy. This energy can eradicate the foci (sites) and electrical pathways that are causing the abnormal rhythm—atrial fibrillation. The procedure is usually effective but is not without its risks and complications. Often those pathways are in the left side of the heart and access to them is not always simple. (See also chapter 3.)

Surgical approaches are available as well, with surgery affording greater access to the heart.

Do all patients with atrial fibrillation need to be brought back to a normal rhythm?

No. Studies have shown that many patients are not bothered by their hearts' being in atrial fibrillation. In these instances the course of patients in terms of longevity and likelihood of a stroke is no worse than in patients who are kept in a normal rhythm through medication. The need for recurrent hospitalization is even decreased in this group when compared with the group that requires medication and multiple electrical cardioversions to maintain a normal rhythm. But patients in atrial fibrillation must remain on an anticoagulant, Coumadin, for a lifetime. If not, they are at risk of sustaining a stroke.

How will the doctor treat my extra heartbeats?

Isolated extra heartbeats are most often innocuous, but at times may be felt by the patient and be a source of concern. The first step is to diagnose what the cause of the extra heartbeats might be. Having ascertained that they are not dangerous, then behavior modification is a good first step. Caffeine, alcohol, and smoking will all exacerbate and increase the likelihood of extra heartbeats. If the extra heartbeats persist in spite of these precipitants being removed, then there are a variety of medications ranging from antiarrhythmics to beta-blockers which can be utilized. However, reassurance often goes a long way when used in conjunction with lifestyle changes.

The doctor said he detected "VT." It sounded serious. Can a drug make it go away?

"VT" stands for ventricular tachycardia, which refers to a rapid, serious rhythm originating from the lower chambers of the heart. If sustained, this can well be fatal.

Your doctor may place a defibrillator in your heart to keep you safe. Or he may choose to use medications alone. We used to use quinidine and pronestyl, but these drugs were poorly tolerated and often dangerous. These days, you may be started on a drug called *amiodarone* (Cordarone). This is a very powerful and effective drug. It can decrease or even eliminate the dangerous heart rhythm. However, in the long term, amiodarone can be a "poison"—damaging the heart, the lungs, the liver, or other organs.[9]

What kind of device did Vice President Cheney have placed in his heart?

According to newspaper reports, Vice President Dick Cheney had a device that is a combined pacemaker/defibrillator inserted in his heart. This device is designed to protect him from either too slow a heart rate—in which case the pacemaker would take over—or from repetitive rapid ventricular arrhythmias—at which point the device would shock the heart back to a normal rhythm.

Does the fact that I have palpitations mean that I will someday require a pacemaker?

No. A pacemaker is recommended when heart block is identified. In this instance a pacemaker is placed so that the heart rate does not fall below the lower limits set for the pacemaker. Palpitations are usually caused not by too slow a pulse from heart block but rather from too fast a pulse or from extra heartbeats. Thus, most patients with palpitations do not ultimately require a pacemaker.

10
RHEUMATIC FEVER, ANEURYSMS, AND CARDIAC TUMORS

RHEUMATIC FEVER

Case 1. Your Author's Girlfriend.

The author was just nineteen, a sophomore in college, when he met Angela. She was beautiful, with long, dark hair, a figure to die for, and an infectious smile. He was just getting to know her. They had had a great date, a fun ride back to her house in the convertible (fortunately none of the spark plugs had fouled, so there had been no roadside repair). The author was about to reach around her shoulder to "get to know her better" when he started to worry about that very "infectious" smile. Angela had told him she had suffered from rheumatic fever when she was fourteen. She had been quite ill at that time, missing two and a half months from school. And, she explained, she now had a heart murmur. She sure looked healthy now—very, very healthy, in fact. He was just about to kiss Angela, that all-important first kiss, when a little voice went off in his head. What is this rheumatic fever? Is it serious? Would it be gone by now? Could it still be lingering? Was she in trouble? And, above all, was it contagious? At that time, kids didn't have AIDS to contend with, but mononucleosis—the so-called kissing disease—was all the rage. Even in those days, young love had not been totally carefree. But Angela was leaning over, she had pursed her lips, and she was closing her eyes. Discretion was thrown to the wind. He decided to kiss first and ask questions later.

Little did the author know, although rheumatic fever was definitely not contagious, years later its eventual ravages on the valves of the heart would form a substantial part of his cardiac surgical practice.

What is rheumatic fever? Is it contagious?

Were your author's fears misplaced? The answer is yes. The infection that causes rheumatic fever occurs decades before the late valve damage. There was absolutely no threat of contagion, despite the intimacy of contact, at the stage of late valve disease.

Rheumatic fever is a disease that represents a reaction of the body to a prior streptococcal infection. Streptococcus is a very common bacterium that can affect the upper respiratory passages and other sites. The initial infection usually presents as a sore throat. The body responds to the streptococcal sore throat with a reaction that may affect the joints, the nervous system, or the heart. If the heart is affected, this is most often manifested by scarring of the heart valves. This may lead to either mitral valve narrowing (mitral stenosis) or leakage (mitral regurgitation). Similarly, the aortic valve may be narrowed (aortic stenosis) or become leaky (aortic regurgitation). Although the antecedent streptococcal sore throat may be contagious, rheumatic fever is not a contagious disease. The offending streptococcus is long gone by the time the valves become scarred. Fortunately, since the advent of penicillin and other antibiotics, the incidence of untreated streptococcal sore throat and consequent rheumatic fever has lessened dramatically in developed countries.

How can I tell if my children or I should see a doctor for a sore throat? We don't want to contract rheumatic fever, but we can't be running to the doctor with every sore throat.

It is better to bring a child into a doctor's office if there is any possibility that a sore throat may be due to a streptococcus. If the child complains of a sore throat and has a high fever, or if the sore throat persists for several days, or if there is a yellowish exudate in the throat, the child should be evaluated by his or her pediatrician. A simple swabbing of the throat and a culture of that swab can result in a diagnosis within twenty-four hours. A nurse or physician assistant can perform this test in minutes. Therefore, the benefits of coming into the office far outweigh the downside. A very small percentage of streptococcal infections go on to cause rheumatic fever, maybe one in many thousands. These days, we tend to treat early, and thus forestall the late sequellae.

ANEURYSMS: AORTIC DISSECTION

What is an aneurysm?

An aneurysm is a swelling of the aorta, the main blood vessel of the body. The aorta begins just above the heart and rises straight up in the front of the chest (*ascending aorta*) toward the top of the body. At that level, it takes a turn, called the *aortic arch*, toward the back

Case 2. The Professor's Wife.

Your surgeon author was out with his kids on a Sunday afternoon. He remembers this vividly, as he was responsible for the children, aged three and five, on this particular day. His wife was off on a rare girls' day out. The beeper buzzed, and Dr. Cohen was on the line. "John, I need you in the ER, and I need you now. A professor's wife is dying. You need to take her to the OR immediately." Dr. Cohen was known for his equanimity and his judgment. This cryptic message from him was significant. The kids were hastily deposited at a neighbor's, and it was off to the ER.

Carmella was twenty-eight years old. Dr. Cohen had followed her for the four years since her husband had come to Yale as an assistant professor in the School of Epidemiology and Public Health. She had Marfan syndrome, an inherited disorder that gave her a tall, thin frame and predis-posed her to diseases of the aorta. Her aorta had been small for an aneurysm, only 4.8 centimeters, not yet in the danger zone. But this condition was unpre-dictable.

Carmella had been home with her husband when she suffered sudden, severe chest pain for the first time in her life. The pain moved along her left chest and down her left flank. She sud-denly became pale and lost consciousness. Her hus-band first called 911, then Dr. Cohen, who was in the ER by the time the ambu-lance arrived.

Dr. Cohen knew right away what was awry. One glimpse was enough for him to know that Carmella, a vibrant social worker, was suddenly very, very sick—clinging to life by a fine thread. When he put his stethoscope to Carmella's chest, he nodded silently to himself. There it was, the murmur of aortic insuffi-ciency—which she had never had before. He knew right away that her aorta had split—what we call an aortic dissection. She had lost consciousness because the aorta had leaked internally into the heart sac, causing shock. Surgery was the only hope.

of the body. From the aortic arch, the aorta runs along the spine all the way down the chest (*descending aorta*), through the diaphragm, and into the abdomen. In the midabdomen (*abdominal aorta*), just opposite the belly button, the aorta splits into two branches, each of which heads off to supply blood to one of the legs. The aorta, normally about 1 to 1-1/2 inches in diameter, gets smaller as it gives off branches in its course toward the lower body.

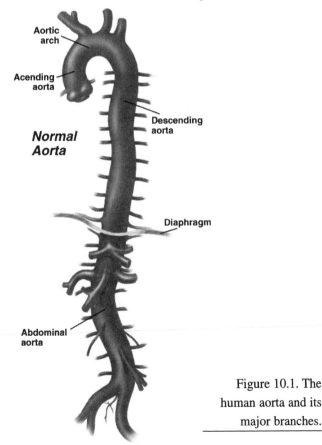

Aortic arch

Acending aorta

Normal Aorta

Descending aorta

Diaphragm

Abdominal aorta

Figure 10.1. The human aorta and its major branches.

The ascending aorta gives off (supplies, as branches) the coronary arteries, which provide blood to the heart muscle itself. The aortic arch gives off all the important branches to the head, brain, and arms. The descending aorta gives off branches to each rib. The abdominal aorta gives off the branches to the liver, intestines, kidneys, and other important internal organs. Finally, each of the terminal branches of the abdominal aorta goes off to one of the legs.

Each major segment of the aorta can develop an aneurysm. Aneurysms of the major segments of the aorta are illustrated in the figure. An aneurysm is a swelling of the aorta, so that the aorta bulges and becomes enlarged. Even the branches of the aorta can, at times, develop aneurysms. Sometimes, these bulges can have a shape reminiscent of the inner tubes that bulged through the wall of old, tube-type automobile tires.

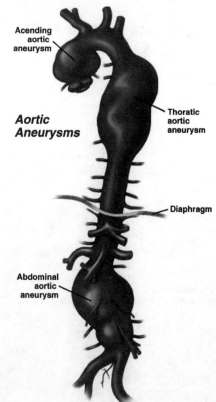

Acending
aortic
aneurysm

*Aortic
Aneurysms*

Thoratic
aortic
aneurysm

Diaphragm

Abdominal
aortic
aneurysm

Figure 10.2.
Aortic
aneurysms.

Why are aneurysms important?

Aneurysms are significant for one simple reason: they can rupture. A ruptured aneurysm often results in fatality, as blood is lost internally into the chest or abdominal cavities. Death can occur very quickly, at times within minutes or even seconds.

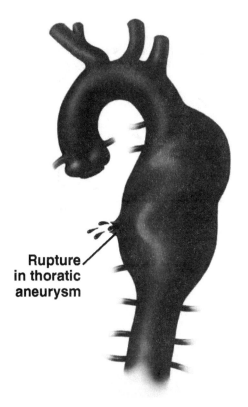

Rupture in thoratic aneurysm

Figure 10.3.
Aneurysm
rupture.

Wouldn't I feel an aneurysm if I had one?

Sometimes, the patient can have pain related to an aneurysm. For an aneurysm of the ascending aorta, the pain is usually felt behind the breastbone. For the descending aorta, the pain is usually felt in the high back, between the shoulder blades. For the abdominal aorta, the pain is usually felt in the lower back or flanks. The pain of an aneurysm is usually a nagging, aching pain, not brought on by any specific activity. Patients can usually differentiate the pain of an aneurysm from the pain felt in muscles, joints, and the spine, but they should consult their physician to help with this differentiation.

Unfortunately, most patients do not feel pain from an aneurysm until the moment it ruptures. That is the reason that detection and preemptive extirpation (removal) are of such importance.

At the specific moment of rupture, the patient feels an extremely severe pain, sharp and sudden. She may lose consciousness from internal bleeding. Death may occur very quickly. Sometimes, the internal layers of body tissues can contain the blood stream temporarily, giving a chance for prompt hospital transfer and surgical treatment.

How can my doctor predict when my aneurysm might rupture?

If your aneurysm is causing pain over a period of time, it is likely that it will rupture. If your aneurysm is growing, it is likely that it will rupture.

Also, if your aneurysm has attained a certain size, we know that the chance of rupture increases. For the ascending aorta, if it grows to six centimeters in diameter, nearly three times the normal size, it is very likely to rupture. Extensive research at Yale University has shown that the chance of rupture or death from an aneurysm is 14 percent per year once the aneurysm attains a size of six centimeters. How big is six centimeters? A soft drink can has a diameter of 6.4 centimeters. So, if your aorta has reached a dimension about that of a soft drink can, you are at significant risk for a rupture.

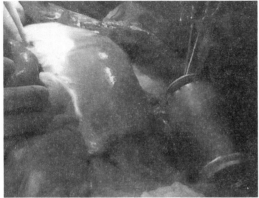

Figure 10.4. A soft drink can next to a large thoraco-abdominal aneurysm. The chest and abdomen have been opened in a single, large incision. The patient's head is to the left of the image shown. An aneurysm this size is in the "red zone" of danger.

What can be done about my aneurysm?

Your aneurysm can be surgically removed and replaced by an artificial graft.

For patients too elderly or too feeble to undergo surgical removal of the aneurysm, internal grafts (called stents) can be delivered by catheter, without a major incision, in an effort to seal off the aneurysm from the bloodstream. This may help to prevent rupture in selected cases. Years of additional experience is needed to know if stent therapy effectively prevents rupture.

What is meant by *aortic dissection*?

Aortic dissection is an internal split within the wall of the aorta. Blood under pressure gets into the wall of the aorta and splits that wall apart. Blood has gained access where it shouldn't be, but it has not—not yet, that is—perforated completely through the wall of the aorta.

This is the condition that affected Carmella in the story at the beginning of this section. Not surprisingly, as the aorta splits internally, the patient feels excruciating, knifelike, tearing pain. This pain is one of the most severe that a human being can ever feel. Aortic dissection, as in Carmella's case, is very serious.

Free rupture of a dissection can occur, leading to death from internal bleeding into a body cavity (pericardium, chest, or abdomen). Blood supply to internal organs can be disrupted by the dissection. In many cases, urgent surgery is required. As in Carmella's case, surgery can save the patient's life.

My doctor told me I have an aneurysm of my heart itself. How can that be?

Up to this point, we have talked about aneurysms of the aorta. Aneurysms can indeed affect the heart itself. If you suffer a transmural, or through-and-through, heart attack, the involved muscle in that zone is dead. In some cases, that dead muscle becomes very thin and, over time, stretches out, producing a bulge very reminiscent of the bulge in an old-fashioned tube tire. You can see this in the following figure.

Now, aneurysms of the heart, unlike those of the aorta, never rupture. We do not know why they behave differently in this respect. However, aneurysms of the heart, of the left ventricle specifically, can cause trouble in a number of ways. They can cause heart failure by distorting the normal size, shape, and contraction pattern of your left ventricle—the vital pumping chamber of your heart. They can allow clots to form inside the bulging area—clots that can travel to dangerous parts of your circulation, such as the brain or the coronary arteries themselves. They can cause arrhythmias, as the neighboring tissue on the border of the aneurysm can be electrically unstable. And aneurysms can cause chest pain. In general, an aneurysm of the left ventricle is a bad thing to have. Outlook for these patients is among the poorest of any group with heart disease.

The good news is that aneurysms of the heart can be removed, usually in conjunction with a coronary artery bypass operation.

Although we cannot restore muscle that has died, by removing the aneurysm we can restore the shape and size of the heart, improving the patient's outlook and preventing many of the complications of an aneurysm. Although it may sound dangerous to remove an aneurysm of the heart and suture and reshape the main pumping chamber, this procedure, since being pioneered by the preeminent heart surgeon Dr. Denton Cooley in 1958, has become quite safe and reproducible today.

Appearance of aneurysm

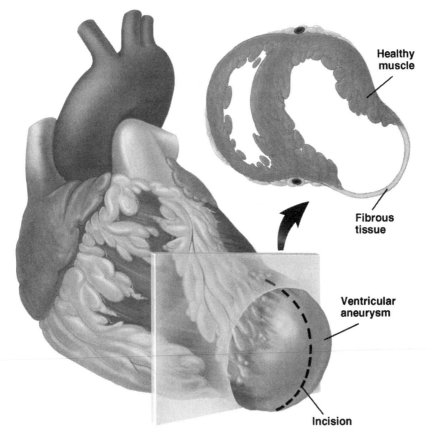

Healthy muscle

Fibrous tissue

Ventricular aneurysm

Incision

Figure 10.5a

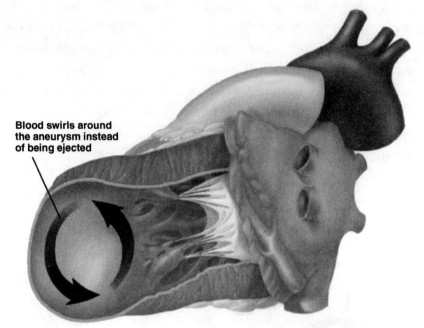

Blood swirls around
the aneurysm instead
of being ejected

Figure 10.5b

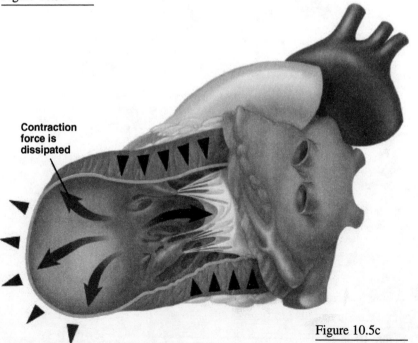

Contraction
force is
dissipated

Figure 10.5c

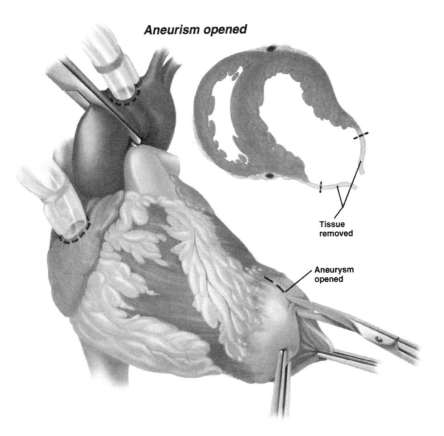

Figure 10.5d

Figures 10.5a, 10.5b, 10.5c, 10.5d, 10.5e, and 10.5f. Left ventricular aneurysm
and its repair. Part a shows the general appearance of a left ventricular
aneurysm. Note the thinning and bulging of the wall of the ventricle, the main
pumping chamber of the heart. Parts b and c depict how the aneurysm hurts
heart function by dissipating the contractile force of the heart into useless
swirling and expanding the aneurysm in systole. Part d shows the aneurysm
being opened at surgery. Part e illustrates the clot (thrombus) that often resides
in the aneurysm (due to stagnation of blood in this area). Part f shows how the
heart is closed after resection of the aneurysm.

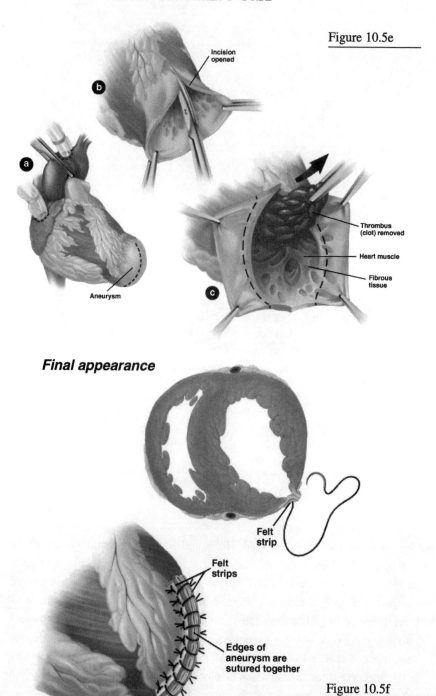

Figure 10.5e

Incision opened

Thrombus (clot) removed

Heart muscle

Fibrous tissue

Aneurysm

Final appearance

Felt strip

Felt strips

Edges of aneurysm are sutured together

Figure 10.5f

Now, for some follow-up on Carmella, the social worker and professor's wife with the acute dissection of her aorta. Your author met her in the ER and took her straight to the operating room. Her aorta and valve were immediately replaced, and she was very sick for several days. She has recovered fully and, over the ensuing ten years, has become a highly respected watercolor artist, whose paintings have been exhibited in New York City and throughout the nation.

CARDIAC TUMORS

Case 3. The Girl from Ipanema.

The distinguished and normally unflappable Dutch cardiologist had grabbed one of the authors, Dr. Elefteriades, by the lapel. Your author was about to leave town for a lecture trip. The morning's operation had been completed, and the patient was safely ensconced in the ICU. Time was short to make the plane.

But Dr. Wackers would not take no for an answer. The patient was a twenty-three-year-old female from Brazil. She was living here with her husband, a graduate student in the Business School.

Selma had been sick for days. She had been shipped over to the University Hospital from the infirmary. Doctors there thought she had mitral stenosis, or narrowing of the mitral valve. So far, it sounded routine, hardly enough to cancel a major trip and justify the urgency of tone in the descriptions. Many of the prominent staff of doctors could oversee her care.

Then came more. The blood pressure was low, very low. Hmm, that wasn't right. The bicarbonate was 5. Had your author heard right—5? No living patient could have a level so low, indicating extreme accumulation of acid in the body. The platelet count was 20—down from a normal 250. That could only indicate a premoribund condition.

Dr. Wackers took your author first to the echo lab. The minute the image came up on the screen, Dr. Elefteriades knew his plans had to change. The tumor filled the left atrium, and with each heartbeat blocked the mitral valve, virtually halting blood flow from the heart.

Orders were given to prepare the operating room, while the team hastened to the emergency room. From afar, your author saw a beautiful young woman, in full makeup and stylishly appointed. Only as the team approached could he make out that she was barely breathing. No pulse was palpable anywhere, not in the arms, not in the neck, and not in the groin. Only with vigorous stimulation did Selma rouse to a momentary consciousness. Dr. Elefteriades had already given the order to prepare the OR. The intern in the emergency department was dismayed that your author was not paying attention to the laundry list of laboratory parameters he was announcing—tests both completed and pending. Your author had other plans in mind. He grabbed the stretcher himself and started running for the elevator. The details of the labs did not really matter. The huge growth had to be removed. It was literally choking her heart to the point of death.

Can the heart ever become affected by tumors or cancer?

Yes, the heart can be prey to tumors. The only type of tumor that is seen with frequency is called an *atrial myxoma*. This tumor often occurs in young people. It usually arises in the left atrium. It produces symptoms when small particles break off, traveling to the brain or other organs. Sometimes the myxoma can interfere with function of the mitral valve, causing shortness of breath. In any case, the diagnosis is made with a cardiac echo exam.

Surgery is required immediately if the myxoma is producing symptoms or looks dangerously sized or positioned. Fortunately, surgery is usually curative. Although this is not a completely benign tumor, it does not usually spread to other parts of the body. After surgery, most patients have every reason to expect to live a long and full life.

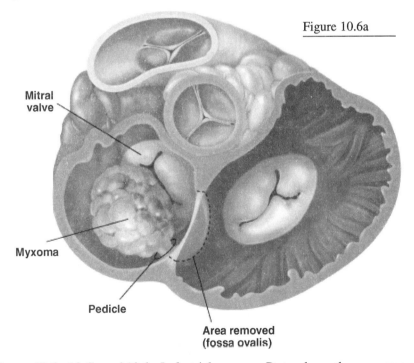

Figure 10.6a

Mitral valve

Myxoma

Pedicle

Area removed (fossa ovalis)

Figures 10.6a, 10.6b, and 10.6c. Left atrial myxoma. Part a shows the appearance of the myxoma with the heart sliced transversely. Part b shows the appearance of the myxoma with the heart sliced longitudinally. Part c shows our surgical approach for removing the myxoma, which must be done very gently so as to avoid shedding particles of the friable myxoma tissue into the bloodstream.

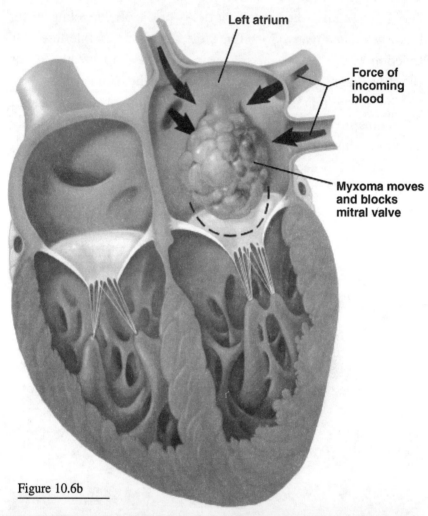

Figure 10.6b

Now, some follow-up on Selma, the young woman from Brazil. We took her straight to the operating room from the ER. As expected, her heart stopped as soon as she was anesthetized—from the poor circulatory state related to the plugging of the mitral valve by her tumor. Moving with enhanced urgency, we put her on the heart-lung

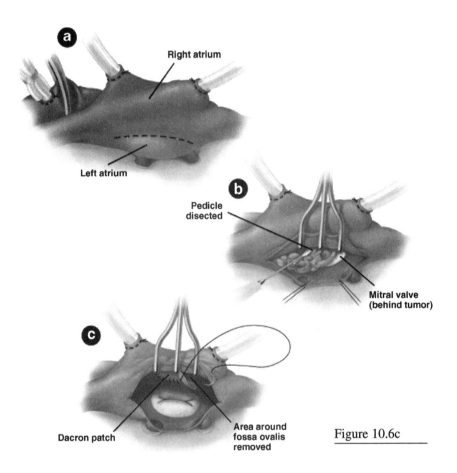

Figure 10.6c

machine, opened the heart, and removed the tumor. A year later, she is fine, absolutely fine. Her husband has finished his studies, and they are returning to Brazil. An echo exam found her heart to be absolutely normal. The author gave her his go-ahead to become pregnant and have her first child. We anxiously await word—and pictures, of course.

Chapter
11
SO YOU NEED HEART SURGERY

(For All Heart Surgery Patients)

T his chapter will discuss general questions concerning cardiac surgery. (Specific questions about particular operations are discussed in separate chapters later in the book.)

How do I prepare for heart surgery?

Many heart operations are required on an urgent basis. In such circumstances, of course, there is not time to prepare in any specific way. However, the vast majority of heart operations can be done in a planned or what we call elective fashion. For these scheduled operations, some preparation is possible.

Most important is that you keep active. We do not want you to arrive deconditioned and debilitated. The body deteriorates very quickly with inactivity. If you remain sedentary in the days or weeks leading up to your surgery, you will find yourself with weaker bones, muscles, and lungs. This weakness will be exacerbated by the changes around the time of your operation. Your recovery will be prolonged and your health will be in jeopardy. So, keep active. In most cases, keep going to work, shopping, driving, walking, even exercising. In unusually severe cases of angina, your doctor may ask that you limit your exertion to activities that do not provoke anginal pain.

If you are seriously overweight, your doctor may allow weeks or even months in scheduling your operation to permit you to lose weight. Even a drop of five or ten pounds will improve your breathing and mobility after an operation and make your recovery quicker and more secure.

Also critical in your preparation: quit smoking. If you arrive at the hospital with your lungs still affected by cigarette smoke, you will be much more prone to bronchitis, pneumonia, and even death after cardiac surgery. If you can arrive with clean lungs, you will recover better and more quickly, as well as more safely. Your general medical doctor can usually help you decrease or stop using cigarettes with one of the many adjuncts now available for this purpose (gums, patches, pills, and the like).

In most cases, stop taking aspirin about two weeks before the scheduled date of your operation. Aspirin thins your blood. This can be a problem at the time of cardiac surgery, when your blood needs to be thick enough so that you do not bleed from surgical sites. Your surgeon will advise you specifically about his preferences. Only in very rare cases with critical blockages in coronary arteries do we advise continuing the aspirin up to the time of surgery. We do have antidotes that can be brought to bear to counteract the aspirin, but we prefer not to expose the patient to these, as they are products from the blood of other human beings. Nonsteroidal anti-inflammatory medications can also affect your blood in the same way as aspirin. Many elderly patients take these drugs for arthritis. Check your list of medications and vitamins carefully and ask your cardiologist, your surgeon, or the anesthesiologist if you have any questions.

The anesthesiologist will advise you regarding other drugs. Most other medications can be continued up to and including the day of surgery. Medications for arrhythmias, for heart failure, and even water pills can usually be continued. The morning of surgery, take only those pills specifically prescribed by the anesthesiologist and/or surgeon, and take them with only a sip of water. You need to have an empty stomach when you reach the operating room. If you do not, the risk from anesthesia will be too great, and your surgery will be cancelled. The reason for this precaution is that if anesthesia is delivered on a full stomach, there is a high probability of food materials getting into your lungs should you vomit, with potentially disastrous consequences. So, have nothing to eat or drink by mouth after midnight the night before surgery, except for the morning pills and the sip of water you need to swallow them.

Critically important is to arrive with a positive attitude and a determination to do well and to recover quickly. Your family can help to achieve and maintain such a positive attitude. This is so important that your authors have many times wished that they could isolate and bottle this "positive attitude" factor, so that it could be distributed to all patients. A patient who is pessimistic and unfocused on recovery and resumption of work and family life is more likely to do poorly.

Your authors remember the case of an octogenarian widower. He arrived for his heart surgery with a twinkle in his eye, as he had recently befriended a "younger woman"—a spry seventy-five-year-old square dancer. We could sense his determination to recover—so that he could resume and advance this romance. We knew his intense motivation would make him do well. He flirted with our nurses, but was well and home within five days of his surgery.

What type of incision will you use for my heart surgery?

Most open heart procedures are done through an incision that we call a *median sternotomy*. This incision is placed in the middle of the front of the chest right over the center of the breastbone, as shown in the following diagram.

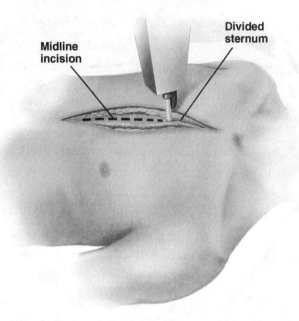

Figure 11.1. The median sternotomy incision. This is done with a sabre saw, like the ones in a home workshop.

Although you may think of this as potentially very painful, it is actually one of the most comfortable incisions used in any type of major surgery. The nerve supply to the chest begins at the back near the spine. Most nerve endings have petered out by the time the nerve fibers reach the center of the chest. This may be one reason why this incision is relatively comfortable. Another reason is that we wire the chest firmly together after the operation is completed, so that there is very little movement of the sides of the breastbone when you breathe or move. The following figure shows an X-ray of a patient who has had open heart surgery. You can see the heavy wires, like paper clips in thickness, which are used to reapproximate the breastbone after surgery. These wires are permanent, but completely inert. You will not be aware of them in any way. And, no, we have not had any patient complain that he has triggered a metal detector at an airport because of his sternal wires.

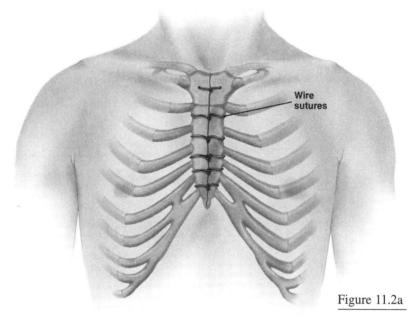

Figure 11.2a

Figure 11.2. Schematic (a) and X-ray (b, front view, c, side view) showing sternal wires.

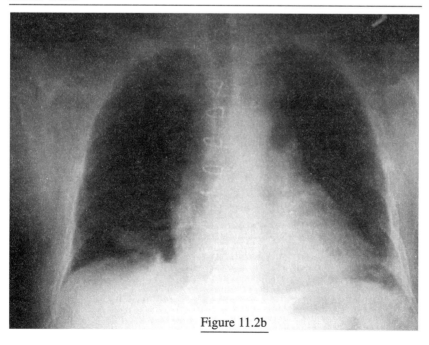

Figure 11.2b

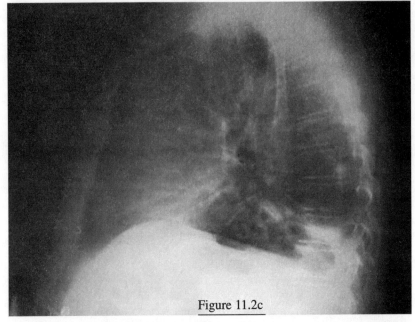

Figure 11.2c

This relative comfort of open heart surgery is in contradistinction to an abdominal incision, for example, for a gallbladder or colon or uterus operation. With such abdominal incisions, every breath moves the muscles of your belly wall, leading to severe pain. Most of our patients liken the pain of the median sternotomy for cardiac surgery to that of a bad toothache. By the end of a week, the discomfort has dissipated considerably. By one month, the pain is nearly gone. For up to a year, however, you may be troubled by your incision on certain days.

What are the sternal wires made of?

The sternal wires are made of a special stainless steel alloy. This material is completely inert vis-à-vis your body's tissues. Unlike most foreign bodies, these wires evoke no irritative effects. Your body is essentially unaware of their presence. We have reoperated decades after these wires were placed, and they appear to be completely brand-new, just like the day they were placed, with no neighboring inflammation or scarring. And, by the way, no, your wires do not rust.

Incidentally, these wires do occasionally break at some point. Your primary doctor may become alarmed and ask you to call your surgeon immediately. As a matter of fact, breaks of these wires that occur a long time after surgery are of absolutely no consequence. This finding on a late X-ray is a curiosity and nothing more. The bone has already healed by that point, and the wires, broken or not, are by then irrelevant.

Don't you need to go in and remove the wires after the breastbone is healed?

No, there is absolutely no need to go in and remove the sternal wires at any point, even if they should be broken. The only time we remove these wires is if they start to poke out against the inside of your skin. This happens very rarely. If this should happen to you, you may feel a very sharp, very localized pain at the site of a sternal wire. Usually, if this is the case, you will be able to feel the sharp edge of a wire if you examine the area with your fingertips. If the associated discomfort is troublesome to you, the offending wire should be removed. This takes literally minutes, under local anesthesia plus sedation. There is no reason for you to tolerate the discomfort of a "poking" wire, which can be severe. Occasionally, you may be able to see some redness or thinning of the skin over the poking wire. These are signs that the wire is about to protrude through the skin. You should not allow this to happen. You should contact your surgeon promptly if it seems that the end of a wire is about to protrude. This may happen even years after the original operation, especially if you have recently lost a large amount of weight, decreasing the amount of fat buffer between your wires and the undersurface, or dermis, of your skin.

How will my pain be treated?

As indicated above, the median sternotomy incision, through which most open heart operations are performed, is a comfortable incision. However, you will have pain. There are many techniques at the disposal of your medical team to keep this pain to a minimum.

The mainstay of early postoperative pain control is still narcotic medications, such as morphine, Demerol, and their related drugs. You will receive some of these drugs through your IV when you are in the intensive care unit following your surgery. Since the drugs are administered via IV, the process is painless. After you graduate to the regular floor, alternate forms of narcotics will be given in pill form. One popular pill, which combines narcotic medication with aspirin, is Percocet. You will probably be started on one pill every four hours. This pill, like other similar narcotic-based oral pain medications, is quite powerful. It may make you dizzy or light-headed. It may make you quite drowsy. If you are small or elderly or frail or completely unused to narcotics, you may have an exaggerated reaction to such medications. Occasionally, certain robust patients may need two pills every four hours.

You should remember that narcotic medications may also cause other side effects. You may feel confused or exhausted. You may even have some hallucinations. Chances are that you will become constipated, as the narcotic medications put your intestines "to sleep."

In the weeks right after surgery, do not hesitate to take your narcotic medications—they are essential to your comfort and well-being. If you allow yourself to become uncomfortable and, consequently, you do not physically move about well, you will be more prone to pneumonia and blood clots. Do not try to be a hero. You need not worry about addiction, which is very unlikely from a brief course of postoperative narcotics.

There are many new medications that were not available even several years ago that are very effective at relieving postsurgical pain without the deleterious effects of narcotics. These new medications include Toradol and, until recently, Vioxx. (Vioxx was taken off the market because of cardiac complications.) These drugs do not make you drowsy or cause you to become dizzy. Often, taking these drugs as baseline therapy permits you to use less narcotic medication.

Most cardiothoracic surgical programs have a formal pain service available for consultation. This team is usually headed by an anesthesiologist who has special training and experience in relief of pain. The team usually includes one or two anesthesia residents and one or two nurses, as well. If your pain should be unusually severe, this team can be called to assist in its management. They will talk to you about how you are feeling and make informed suggestions to your surgical team.

You should take the narcotics as often as necessary (within guidelines) during the early days after the operation. Do not try to be a hero. You will actually impede your recovery severely if you allow untreated pain to limit the depth of your breathing or to discourage you from getting up and walking. You will even need to take some of the narcotic pills home with you for use at times when the pain is especially severe. Over the first one or two weeks after discharge, you will find that extra-strength Tylenol comes to suffice for your pain control. In another week or two, you will no longer need any pain medication.

How long will my breastbone take to heal?

Healing of bone or any other wound or tissue proceeds at the same rate—the rate of formation of collagen, the structural protein of all our body tissues. Healing is, generally, 50 percent complete by sixty days after surgery. In practical terms, the strength of your breastbone will be so great by three months that you can do, or lift, anything you desire. Even after one month has passed, it is very unlikely that you will do anything to impair the healing of the bone.

Is there anything I need to watch for in regard to the healing of my breastbone?

You do need to watch for signs of infection or instability of your breastbone after median sternotomy.

Infection would usually manifest itself by way of multiple symptoms. You may notice severe or increasing redness around the wound. You may notice swelling, like a large pustule forming at some point in the wound. You may develop drainage from the wound, which may be cloudy or, to use the medical term, *purulent*. There may be associated fever or a general feeling of not being well, which we call *malaise*. These would all be signs of potential infection, which would clearly merit your being seen promptly by your surgeon or his team.

Deep infection of the breastbone is potentially very serious, even life-threatening. If you report your symptoms and seek attention promptly, chances are that this infection can be treated appropriately and definitively, returning you to normal and long life. Diabetics are more prone than others to infection of the breastbone, but, still, this occurs in fewer than 4 percent of open heart cases.

Instability is felt by virtue of relative movement of the right and left hand portions of the breastbone. You may even be able to feel a click, sometimes a painful one, upon certain movements or in assuming certain positions. This can indicate that the wires have broken or torn through your breastbone. This is different from infection but can lead to infection by allowing bacteria to gain access to the space under the breastbone called the *mediastinum*.

You will feel numbness around your chest incision; this reflects the interruption of microscopic nerves in the territory by the incision itself. Some of this numbness will resolve and some of it will persist but be forgotten later. The numbness itself is no cause for concern.

You may also feel a band of numbness (or pain) just to the left of your breastbone, corresponding to the area where the left internal mammary artery was harvested. We actually cauterize the mammary artery and its fascia (its membranelike covering) and accompanying nerves and veins out of its bed on the inside of your chest wall. It is not at all surprising that patients feel pain along the site of this surgical manipulation or that that part of the chest feels numb for weeks or months.

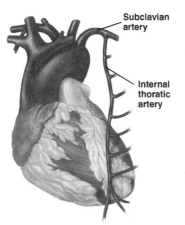

Subclavian artery

Internal thoratic artery

Figure 11.3. Mammary pedicle take-down (harvesting) and corresponding area of numbness. The pedicle is the strip of tissue that surrounds the internal mammary artery. This tissue is harvested along with the delicate artery. The top figure shows where the mammary artery (also called the internal thoracic artery) lies. The bottom figure shows how we mobilize this (by electrocautery) from the inside of the chest wall. You will have an area of pain and numbness corresponding to this strip of tissue to the left of your breastbone while you are recovering from your CABG.

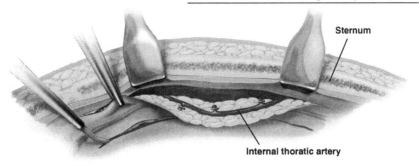

Sternum

Internal thoratic artery

You will also feel numbness along your leg incision due to a similar interruption of microscopic nerve endings. Also, you may feel numbness near the inner part of your ankle because of manipulation of the saphenous nerve, which provides sensation to the skin of your lower leg but runs precisely along the saphenous vein that we harvest. Such ankle numbness is also no cause for concern. The numbness will resolve and become the new "normal" way that you feel. Your brain will soon forget about this—as it does in most such situations in which numbness persists over time.

What if I do develop an infection in my wound? What happens then?

If you develop an infection of your leg wound, you will, of course, receive some antibiotics, either through IV or in the form of pills. Often, we need to open a portion of the leg incision in cases of infection. We take out a few stitches or staples to allow any pus to escape. We then leave that portion of the wound open.

The open portion of the wound is treated by packing it with a gauze soaked in a local antibacterial solution two to four times daily. One popular solution is actually made by diluting Clorox solution in sterile saline. This is called Dakin's Solution. We usually use it in a half-strength or quarter-strength form. Over time, usually four to eight weeks, nature will—believe it or not—close this wound herself. In medical parlance this is called *closure by secondary intention.* The process is accomplished in two ways: Nature causes the open area to shrink; this is called *wound contraction.* And nature causes new skin to grow toward the center of the wound; this is called *re-epithelialization.* In order for the re-epithelialization to occur, the bed of tissue in the open wound must transform to what we call healthy *granulation tissue.* This is beefy, red tissue that the body grows to fill the gap in the skin and to provide a healthy bed of clean tissue. An open wound does not get infected because it is intrinsically protected by the fact that it drains freely to the outside. These wounds do not generally need to be treated sterilely; clean, nonsterile treatment suffices.

Periodically, your surgeon or another medical staff member will perform a surgical cleansing, called *debridement*, in which devitalized skin or tissue is removed by using a scalpel. This is not painful at all, as the devitalized tissue is devoid of active nerve endings.

It is fairly safe to say that we have never heard of anyone who died from a problem with an incision on the leg. These wounds can be a nuisance for weeks, occasionally months, but, eventually, they will close, with no lasting adverse impact on your health—if they are treated properly.

Also, the recent advent of endoscopic harvesting of the saphenous vein—which is done minimally invasively using a lighted scope through a tiny incision—has nearly eliminated the incidence of leg wound infections as a complication of the coronary artery bypass procedure.

If the sternotomy wound should get infected, that represents a problem of a greater magnitude. In rare cases, the infection is only very superficial, and it can be treated by opening and applying dressings as described above.

More often, however, when the chest incision does become infected, the deeper layers, including the breastbone, are involved. This is usually treated by a plastic surgical revision of your wound, using "flaps" of muscle borrowed from nearby areas. Although infection of the median sternotomy can be life-threatening, this treatment usually suffices, with no long-term major sequellae.

What is heparin?

Heparin is another type of blood thinner. It is a very powerful drug. This is the drug that we give in the operating room to prevent blood clots while you are on the heart-lung machine.

Heparin is an intravenous drug; that is, we give it by injection into your IV.

Unlike Coumadin, heparin works immediately and wears off quickly (within hours). For this reason, it is very helpful in the hospital setting. You may be placed on heparin temporarily while your Coumadin level is building to the desired range.

What does the term *open heart surgery* mean?

It is understandable that the public may not have a very clear sense of the meaning of the term *open heart surgery*, as even among physicians this wording does not have a single, distinct connotation.

In the strictest sense, open heart surgery refers to those cardiac surgical procedures performed after opening the chambers of the heart. Examples of such procedures are the replacement of heart valves, the extirpation (removal) of aneurysms of the heart, and the closure of abnormal, usually congenital, intracardiac openings ("holes in the heart").

Another meaning of open heart surgery is surgery done with the use of the heart-lung machine (see fig. 11.5). This broadens the connotation of the term to include the common coronary bypass operation. Since the coronary arteries run on the surface of the heart, these operations do not require formally opening the chambers of the heart. Nonetheless, these are substantial heart procedures done with the aid of the heart-lung machine and commonly classed among "open heart" operations.

Do you actually take my heart out of my body?

No, we do not actually take your heart out of your body. Surgical techniques are designed to permit working on all parts of the inside and outside of your heart without its removal.

Only in the case of heart transplantation do we actually remove your heart. In such a case, your old diseased heart is removed in favor of your new, strong one.

What is the heart-lung machine?

For most operations on your heart, the heart must be stopped, either to provide a still, bloodless field conducive to working on the surface of the heart, or to permit opening the heart chambers themselves for internal manipulations to be performed.

When the heart is stopped, its function of propelling the blood to all the organs must be replaced in some way. Otherwise, all the organs would suffer from lack of blood and oxygen and would die slowly. In the very earliest days of cardiac surgery, innovators used cross-circulation by connecting a patient's circulation to that of a loved one, whose heart pumped for both individuals during short periods when the sick patient's heart was being repaired. Figure 11.4 shows such a pioneering procedure being performed in 1955 by the great and controversial innovator Dr. C. Walter Lillehei. Such cross-circulation quickly became obsolete, as technical advances in cardiac surgery blossomed.

In the ensuing years, mechanical systems have been developed that can fully replace the function of the heart and lungs. These systems involve both an artificial heart and an artificial lung, thus the designation "heart-lung machine." The accompanying photographs show the heart-lung machine with the operator, or "perfusionist," at her post in front of the machine.

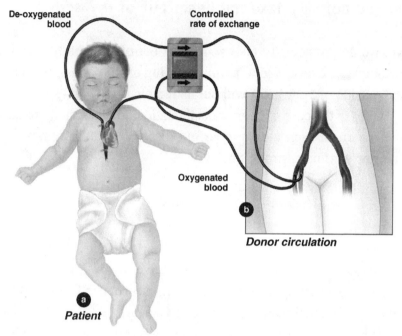

Figure 11.4. Heart surgery pioneer C. Walter Lillehei's historic "cross-perfusion" experiment. Pressurized blood from a parent was used to provide blood flow to the infant undergoing heart surgery.

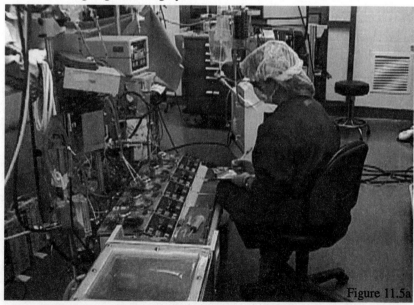

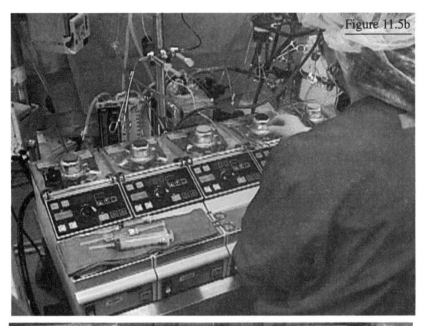

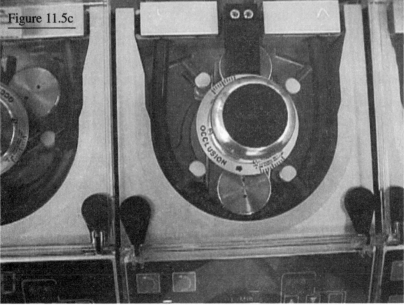

Figures 11.5a, 11.5b, and 11.5c. Heart-lung machine. Parts a and b show the heart-lung machine in use. Part c shows how the roller pump gently squeezes the tubing to propel the blood without traumatizing the red blood cells.

The mechanical function of pumping the blood is served by what is called a *roller pump*. This propels the blood in a very gentle fashion by squeezing a clear, garden hose–sized tubing in which the blood circulates. This method is much less traumatic to the blood cells than if they were propelled by a standard mechanical pump like the water pump in your car.

The function of the lungs is replaced by a canisterlike device in which blood flows slowly and gently over a membrane that has oxygen on the other side. In this way, the blood can pick up oxygen, just as it does in the natural lungs. This oxygen will then be delivered to the body when the blood is propelled back into the body.

How is the heart stopped?

The heart is stopped by perfusing, or supplying, it with a cold salt-water–type fluid containing a high concentration of the mineral potassium. This fluid is called *cardioplegia*, which literally means "heart paralyzer." The potassium stops the electrical activity of the heart by paralyzing the natural electrical pacemaker inside your heart. The cold fluid (ice-cold, in fact) protects the heart muscle, since the colder a body organ becomes, the less oxygen it requires.

The cold fluid is less than 4 degrees Celsius (39.2 degrees Fahrenheit). We aim to keep your heart less than 10 degrees Celsius (50 degrees Fahrenheit) at all times when we have the aorta clamped to perform delicate external or internal work to repair your heart.

How do you restart my heart?

When blood flow is restored to your heart, the potassium-rich cardioplegia solution is washed out, allowing the heart to "wake up"

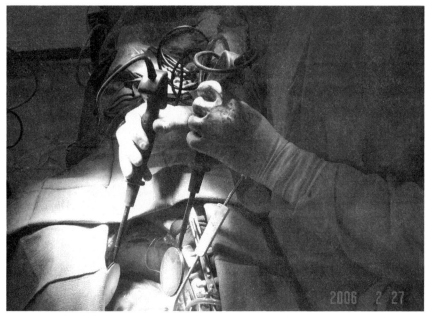

Figure 11.6. Defibrillation paddles.

from its earlier deliberate paralysis. The heart usually begins to beat slowly and then speeds up gradually over a few minutes. Sometimes, depending on the rhythm with which the heart resumes, the heart may be "shocked" back into a regular heartbeat with a strong electrical current delivered directly onto the surface of the heart via electrical "paddles." This is depicted in the accompanying photograph. This is a completely customary and very safe procedure. Occasionally, the heart is paced by temporary wires attached to the surface of the heart until it resumes its normal electrical patterns.

Is the heart-lung machine safe?

The heart-lung machine has been developed, modified, and improved continuously over many decades. It is now, and has been for many years, a supremely reliable and effective mechanical apparatus. It is used millions of times worldwide each year. It is, in fact, a very safe modality of treatment. The heart-lung machine very effectively substitutes for your own heart and lungs while the critical phases of your heart operation are in progress.

How long can I stay on the heart-lung machine?

Most common heart operations, including coronary artery bypass grafting and valve replacement, can be completed with less than two hours on the heart-lung machine. Many preparations are done during surgery before and after the heart-lung machine interval to keep this time to a minimum. The heart-lung machine is very safe for such intervals of time. Essentially all known cardiac operations can be completed within three hours of so-called pump time. This is probably the limit of the totally safe interval for the heart-lung machine. Beyond such intervals, certain negative consequences of being "on bypass" begin to accumulate. These include gradual adverse impacts on the kidneys, lungs, and brain. These adverse effects do not become severe, in general, until bypass times of three, four, or five hours, which are almost unheard of in the present day.

What is "clamp time"?

"Clamp time" refers to a portion of the total bypass time, specifically the time during which blood flow to the heart is "clamped" to permit the most critical portion of the cardiac work to be performed. For example, the connection of bypass grafts to the coronary arteries is done during the "clamp time." Likewise, the actual implantation of a new heart valve is done during the "clamp time." The remainder of the time on the heart-lung machine, before and after the clamp time, is used for less critical portions of the procedure, during which the heart can be allowed to have blood flow without the clamping of the aorta.

It is the cold cardioplegia solution mentioned above that allows the heart to "rest" safely during the clamp time. Clamp times of three hours or so are completely safe (in almost all instances). Almost all cardiac operations can be accomplished during such an interval. If, for some reason, intervals somewhat longer than that are required, the heart gradually accumulates some adverse impact. This adverse impact, which may require medications to restore pumping strength (see below), is usually temporary, resolving within twelve to twenty-four hours. Still longer clamp times may incur unrecoverable injury to the heart muscle.

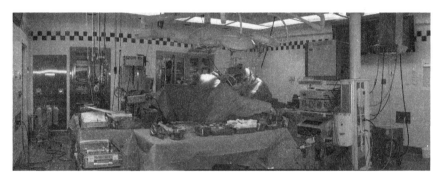

Figure 11.7. Overall OR scene montage.

How many people are in the room while my open heart operation is being performed?

There are four teams involved in your open heart surgery. These teams work in close concert to provide the intricate coordination necessary for the operation. The four teams are surgery, anesthesia, nursing, and perfusion.

Your surgeon will require one or two surgical assistants at the table with him. One will assist him directly from across the table. In the case of the coronary artery bypass procedure, another assistant may remove a vein from your leg. The assistant may be a surgical colleague from your surgeon's group or a physician's assistant (PA), a paramedical professional with extensive training and, in this case, specialized experience in assisting in cardiac surgery. In university medical centers, the assistant may be a resident surgeon. These individuals have usually completed comprehensive training in general surgery and are obtaining additional subspecialized experience in cardiac surgery. These residents are very experienced and mature physicians, usually in their early to midthirties or beyond, before they are assigned the responsibility of assisting at cardiothoracic operations.

An anesthesiologist will be with you throughout the procedure. Her responsibility is to place all the IV lines and tubes required to monitor and treat your heart and lungs during the operation. In many institutions, the anesthesiologist has specialized training in caring for cardiac patients exclusively. She will often be assisted by a nurse anesthetist or resident anesthesiologist. The anesthesiologist is a vital member of the team, whose consultative opinions will be of great importance in your care.

There will generally be two nurses in the room. A *scrub nurse* will be sterilely attired at the table and will hand sutures and instruments to the doctor as necessary. Such individuals are extremely important and highly skilled. By anticipating what will be required, scrub nurses can greatly enhance the conduct of the operation. The *circulating nurse* is not scrubbed at the table. He is free to move about the room and hand supplies to the scrub nurse at the table and to provide communication with the blood bank or the laboratories. He also meters medications that may be required on the table. Because of these many responsibilities, the circulating nurse is a registered nurse, whereas the scrub nurse may be either a registered nurse or a specially trained technician. The scrub nurse and circulating nurse must work as a team for the efficient conduct of the operation to be facilitated.

The perfusionist is another valued and valuable member of the team. He will run the heart-lung machine that supports your circulation during the most critical phase of the procedure. These individuals are not physicians, but they have extensive training in their specialized field. They work in concert with the surgeon and the anesthesiologist in making a myriad of adjustments depending on your vital signs and conditions at various phases of the procedure. The perfusionist is usually supported by a second perfusionist (safety in redundancy) or a perfusion assistant, who may draw and test various blood samples and prepare other mechanical devices that may be required.

How will I feel when I wake up from my operation? Will I feel like I can't breathe?

First and foremost, you do not have to be afraid of waking up or having pain during the operation. You will be anesthetized by medications given through your IV before any incision is made. (Some of the IV placements may be done before you are put to sleep, while you are under heavy sedation.) You will not feel any pain. You will not wake up until the operation is over. Very rarely, a patient can recall events or parts of the conversations that took place during his operation, but always as in a dream state, never with a recollection of pain.

When you do resume consciousness, you will be in the ICU. You may have some pain, but the most discomfort will be from the breathing tube in your windpipe. This tube cannot be removed before you are quite fully awake, because otherwise you would not be able to breathe on your own. Most people feel a gagging sensation from this tube. People vary in their sensitivity. Most are able to relax and cooperate with the nurse in demonstrating their breathing capacity, so that the tube can be removed. The ICU nurse will be right there with you. She will have been watching your body's functions and anticipating your awakening. The nurse is an expert at managing patients through this phase of the recovery. She will keep the uncomfortable interval to the minimum safe period of time. As soon as she confirms that you are conscious and able to breathe for yourself, she will remove the tube. This will provide you considerable relief from discomfort. The nurse will then orient you. Many patients are not even aware that the operation has been performed and that they are recovering; they may think that the operation is yet to come. Your nurse will explain everything that you need to do to contribute to a safe recovery. You should not move excessively to avoid dislodging lines and tubes. You need to cough and breathe deeply as your nurse instructs, to keep your lungs clear. You will probably feel thirsty (because your mouth will be very dry), but the nurse will wait a half hour or more before giving you anything by mouth. She needs to be sure that your throat has recovered from the irritation of the breathing tube before giving you liquids, otherwise there is danger that what you drink may go down the wrong tube—into your lungs rather than down your esophagus (swallowing tube).

Is open heart surgery dangerous?

Heart surgery is not without risk. However, heart surgery has become very, very safe—much safer than when it was first practiced in the 1950s, 60s, and 70s. Open heart surgical procedures are among the most commonly performed operations worldwide. About four hundred thousand coronary bypass procedures are performed in this country yearly; an equal number are performed in the rest of the world. Hundreds of thousands of valve operations are performed here as well. The vast majority of patients recover quickly and without major complications, going on to lead a better-quality life of long duration.

What is the likelihood that I could die during open heart surgery?

The biggest risk, of course, is death. The risk of death for coronary bypass operations for good-risk candidates is about 1 percent to 2 percent. For valve replacement, it is about 3 percent to 4 percent. The good-risk candidate is not of advanced age (less than seventy-five years old), with no extensive prior damage from heart attacks, no severe diabetes, no prior stroke, no severe lung disease, no kidney failure, and not excessively overweight. The vast majority of patients fall in this category. For patients with some or all of these conditions, the risks will be higher. Even in such cases, however, the risk of dying during or after surgery will be no higher than 5 percent to 10 percent. Only the very, very compromised patient will exceed these risk levels.

Could I suffer brain damage from heart surgery?

The next major risk of open heart surgery is stroke. Stroke refers to damage to the brain, usually from lack of blood flow beyond a blockage in a small brain artery or from an embolus, or particle, traveling to and blocking a brain artery. Strokes, of course, can occur naturally, outside the context of heart surgery. But heart surgery can bring on strokes. Blood flow to the brain is more precarious during heart surgery than before or afterward. Also, the manipulations inherent in cardiac operations can dislodge particles, especially pieces of arteriosclerotic material, from the heart into the brain. In general, the risk of stroke is about 1 percent to 2 percent for good-risk coronary artery bypass patients. For valve surgery patients, because the heart itself is opened, increasing the potential for embolism, the risk of stroke is 2 percent to 4 percent. Patients of advanced age or those with prior stroke or disease of the carotid arteries are more vulnerable to stroke. The risk of stroke may be as high as 8 percent to 12 percent in such patients. Strokes may be mild, with minimal impairment, or they may be severe, with weakness of an arm or a leg, or even brain death. Almost invariably, some, often substantial, improvement occurs with rehabilitation, via effort and time. Almost everyone knows of an elderly patient who has fought back bravely from a stroke.

Could I suffer a heart attack during surgery?

A heart attack can occur during surgery. This happens about 5 percent of the time. There are many reasons for this. A bypass graft can close. The feasible bypasses may be insufficient. An embolism to your heart muscle can occur. A bad rhythm of your heart can develop. These heart attacks are usually transient, and good recovery most commonly ensues. The heart may be supported with *inotropic*, or stimulating, medications given through your IV until it becomes stronger. In some cases, a *balloon pump* may be placed to support your struggling heart mechanically (see section below titled "What in the world is a 'balloon' pump?"). In advanced cases, the heart attack can cause *pump failure*, in which your heart cannot support the burden of circulation. If the pump failure is severe or prolonged, it can threaten your life and can even be fatal.

What other risks do I need to know about?

As is intuitively obvious, bleeding is a risk of cardiac surgery. These days, with technical and drug advances, however, bleeding is not nearly as common as it used to be. In fact, up to half of all patients do not receive a blood transfusion. The use of transfusion depends not only on the amount of blood lost but also on the starting level of the *hematocrit*, or blood count. In about 4 percent of cases, the patient needs to be returned to the operating room because of excess bleeding, which is apparent from the measured blood drainage collected via the chest tubes left inside the chest. Up to one hundred cubic centimeters per hour is considered normal. If drainage exceeds this level for a prolonged period, we usually "re-explore." This re-exploration operation is usually quick and well tolerated. Often bleeding may have stopped by the time the chest is reopened to check the surgical sites. Just removing collected blood and clots from around the heart can improve heart function. Occasionally, an additional stitch may be placed to supplement the dozens of stitches already in place. These days, it is very rare for a patient to die from bleeding, although this still does occur, sometimes suddenly, even today. Generally, once the patient has made it through the first night after surgery, the danger of bleeding has passed. By that time, nature has largely healed over the connections made by your surgical team.

Respiratory failure, or inability of the lungs to function properly, can occur after surgery. This is seen almost exclusively in those patients with severe preexisting damage to their lungs, usually from smoking. This type of respiratory failure may require a period, sometimes prolonged, on the breathing machine. This type of problem can even be fatal in severely compromised patients.

Infections can occur after surgery. These may affect the lungs (pneumonia) or the urinary tract (UTI, or urinary tract infection). These are usually easily and effectively treated by antibiotics. Occasionally, a bloodstream infection can occur from bacteria traveling along the large IV lines used during and after surgery. This also can be treated effectively, especially by removing the offending IV line. The leg incisions used to harvest your veins for the coronary artery bypass operation can quite frequently become infected. This is usually just a nuisance rather than a life-threatening problem. Antibiotics and local care correct this. On rare occasions, the chest incision itself can become infected. This occurs in about 2 percent to 4 percent of cases. Diabetics are especially vulnerable. Some cases respond to antibiotics, but many may need another plastic surgical operation to bring about complete healing of the wound. Infections of the median sternotomy incision can be both debilitating and life-threatening. Unfortunately, they are not fully preventable.

Kidney failure can occur after surgery, since the operation puts quite a strain on the kidneys. This can be life-threatening. This problem is seen almost exclusively in patients of extremely advanced age who had severely impaired kidney function to start.

It is quite common to have numbness in three fingers of one hand—the little finger and its two adjacent neighbors. This occurs from stretching of the *brachial plexus*, or nerve bundle to the hand. This bundle may be stretched by the simple process of retracting the two sides of the breastbone to gain access to your heart. This problem usually resolves completely within six to twelve months.

An almost infinite list of other potential problems due to cardiac surgery can be defined. These other problems, however, are rare. One of our teachers referred to these as the "imponderables" that may occur from the sheer magnitude and complexity of the operation and of the human organism. You and your family should be aware that unexpected events can occur.

It is important to realize that all the risks enumerated above are not really additive, but overlapping. That is, you do not need to add the risk of death, of stroke, of infection, and so on, to get an overall risk figure. These figures overlap; that is, the patient with a severe stroke may die, so she would be listed in both sets of figures. In simple terms, your overall chance of doing very well with cardiac surgery—without death, stroke, or major other permanent impairment—is probably better than or equal to 95 percent. Only selected high-risk patients would exceed this risk level.

Will I need a blood transfusion?

We take tremendous precautions to preserve your own blood during cardiac surgery. Essentially all blood shed into the incision is harvested and returned to the heart-lung machine itself or to a "cell-saver" device, which spins the blood in a centrifuge to concentrate the red blood cells; these are then returned to you through your IV.

In the OR, we often administer drugs that improve the clotting function of the blood cells in order to minimize bleeding after an operation. Amicar and Aprotinin are trade names of two such popular drugs. The availability of these medications has had a major impact on preventing bleeding following cardiac surgery, especially for complex or reoperative procedures.

Also, we very often continue the conservation of blood by collecting and returning to you the blood that collects from your chest drains after you have returned to the ICU. We call this *autotransfusion*.

Yet, despite all these techniques, not all blood that is shed can be collected and saved, and some patients need blood transfusions during or following cardiac surgery. About 50 percent of patients undergoing cardiac surgery do receive a blood transfusion. The likelihood of your needing a blood transfusion depends predominantly on two factors: the amount of blood lost during and after the operation and the starting blood count.

The blood count is measured in the parameter called the *hematocrit*. A normal hematocrit is 40 to 50 percent. This is measured as a percentage, because it designates the fraction of your blood volume that is made up of solid red blood cells (in contradistinction to the liquid portion of your blood, called the *plasma*. If your hematocrit is good before surgery, you can usually tolerate the certain loss of blood during surgery. Your blood count may still be satisfactory after surgery.

We used to aim to keep the hematocrit above 30 percent after surgery. Today, we have relaxed this criterion somewhat. We are usually content with a postoperative hematocrit of 26 percent or more. The minimum criterion varies depending on the patient. If you are young, have a strong heart, and have no major disease in the arteries supplying blood to your brain, we may even accept a hematocrit of 20 to 22 percent. If you are older, have a weak heart, and have some blockages in the arteries supplying blood to your brain, we may aim for a hematocrit of 30 percent. The higher the hematocrit, the more easily the blood pumped by your heart delivers oxygen to your tissues.

How safe is the blood supply?

Those facilities that monitor and maintain US blood supply have responded extremely well to the challenges of the last several decades. Testing of the blood is extremely thorough and effective. The blood is examined for the HIV virus as well as for hepatitis (types A, B, and C) and other diseases. We have been informed by the blood bank system that the risk of transmitting HIV via blood transfusion is about one in three hundred thousand units of blood transfused. This is a relatively small number. This number is dwarfed by the other risks inherent in your cardiac operation (such as the risk of death and the risk of stroke).

Most patients readily accept the idea of having a transfusion if their team deems it may be necessary. For those who remain reluctant, mechanisms are available to harvest your own blood (auto donation) or the blood of family members (directed donation) prior to the operation. Several provisos apply, however. Only certain patients can safely donate their own blood. Patients with certain types of heart valve disease actually have expanded blood volume and can safely donate. However, angina patients may need each and every blood cell to deliver oxygen to the heart muscle, and they may not be cleared to donate their own blood. Auto donation, when permitted, is done weeks in advance, so that the patient's body has time to replenish its blood store. This, of course, rules out auto donation for patients requiring emergency surgery.

For directed donation from family members, certain restrictions also apply. The blood must be of a compatible blood type. The process takes about five working days, so, again, this is not an option for emergency operations. The blood of your family will be tested for HIV and hepatitis, just as ordinary donated blood would be.

The fact is that five or ten years ago, many patients availed themselves of auto or directed donation. We have seen a declining interest in these modalities in recent years, as the safety of the regular blood supply has been documented.

Of course, although we would use the auto- or directed-donation units of blood first and preferentially, certain patients may need more than one or two units of blood; these additional units would come from the regular blood supply.

What about Jehovah's Witness patients?

Jehovah's Witness patients have very strong moral and clinical issues with receiving blood transfusions. As a rule, surgeons respect these preferences to the letter.

Some cardiac surgeons may decline to operate on Jehovah's Witness patients. Others accept or even encourage these patients to come to them.

The bottom line is that, without the option to transfuse blood, the risks of surgery escalate dramatically. We have watched patients die from bleeding when they could have been saved by blood transfusion—but we were bound by our respect for these patients' moral principles.

In the circumstance of a Jehovah's Witness requiring cardiac surgery, the patient, his family, and the physician team will have a detailed discussion and reach agreement about the patient's wishes and what will and will not be done during and after the operation. If both parties understand and accept the stipulated terms, cardiac surgery proceeds.

Tell me about noninvasive heart surgery.

Heart surgery is inherently major surgery that simply cannot be performed without major impact on the patient. That said, it is true that techniques to minimize the impact, or *invasiveness*, of heart surgery have been developed, especially within the last ten years.

Noninvasive or *minimally invasive* with respect to heart surgery usually means that the operation is done via smaller incisions or without the heart-lung machine. We will describe both.

In the mid-1990s, surgeons began to explore doing open heart surgery through alternate incisions smaller than the median sternotomy incision described previously. One of the most highly publicized procedures was the performance of a coronary artery bypass procedure (usually a single bypass) through a small incision between the fourth and fifth ribs to the left of the breastbone. Similar small incisions between the ribs were also used on occasion for valve surgery. These exploratory forays into alternate incisions to the median sternotomy were driven not only by concerns for the patient but also by powerful market forces: hospitals wanted to offer the latest, cutting-edge technologies to put them one step above their competitors. Surgeons have now found that we were in some ways reinventing the wheel. More experienced surgeons could have told us what they already knew: that the alternate small

incisions between the ribs were actually more painful than the sternotomy incision they were intended to replace! Whenever the space
between ribs, the so-called intercostals space has been entered and
spread, discomfort is felt with each breath during the postoperative
recovery. No such violation of the intercostals space is occasioned
with the traditional median sternotomy incision. Also, surgery
through the smaller incisions was more difficult and less safe than
through the traditional incision. Enthusiasm for these alternate incisions is now fading, and many surgeons have returned enthusiasti-
cally to the traditional median sternotomy incision. Occasionally, a
partial sternotomy incision is used, leaving the very top or the very
bottom of the sternum intact. Even this is not conclusively superior
to the traditional full incision. The bottom line is that the traditional
median sternotomy incision is safe, quick, and comfortable. Our
surgical forebears could have told us this, as they had started open
heart surgery through rib space incisions, and dropped that technique like the proverbial hot potato when the median sternotomy
was discovered.

The authors wish to note that there is still considerable vari-
ability in the incisional approaches at specific institutions. Some
hospitals and surgeons may still offer alternate incisions, with good
results. If this is the case, they will explain their individual preferences and recommendations to you.

Are there benefits to avoiding the heart-lung machine?

The other aspect of minimally invasive heart surgery has to do with
avoiding the heart-lung machine. The heart-lung machine, although
we have described it as a very proven, safe modality, is not without
consequences. In fact, going on the heart-lung machine triggers a virtual explosion of biologic events, which are depicted in figure 11.8.

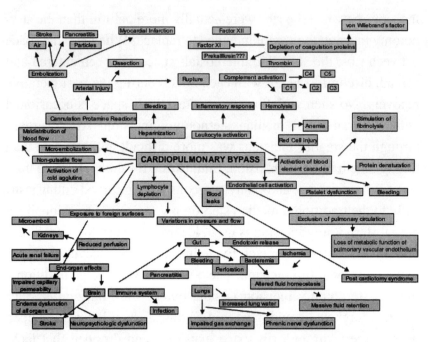

Figure 11.8. Consequences of cardiopulmonary bypass on the heart-lung machine. You can see the virtual "explosion" of the body's reactions to the heart-lung machine. Most of these are very well tolerated.

What the medical terms in that schematic diagram tell us is that the heart-lung machine elicits immunologic reactions (like mild allergic events), that it stimulates many hormones, and that the blood cells are quite affected, among other consequences. Although the schematic depiction seems daunting in terms of potential consequences, the simple fact is that the great majority of patients tolerate these events associated with cardiopulmonary bypass perfectly well. Most patients cannot feel any of these alterations. All these alterations quickly revert to normal within hours, or at most, within days, of the open heart surgery.

For a minority of patients, these events and the consequences of the heart-lung machine can be more severe. The most feared adverse consequence of the heart-lung machine is the liberation of debris from the aorta to the brain, which can cause a stroke. This can happen in a variety of ways. Just placing the cannula (tube) from the heart-lung machine into the aorta may dislodge debris from the aortic wall. The blood flowing from the nozzle of the cannula during bypass can dislodge debris by a "power spray" effect, like that of a high-pressure spray hose.

Most patients do not harbor extensive debris inside the aorta and are not especially vulnerable to this type of problem. In fact, only about 1 to 2 percent of patients suffer a stroke after coronary artery bypass surgery. Patients at most risk are the elderly or those

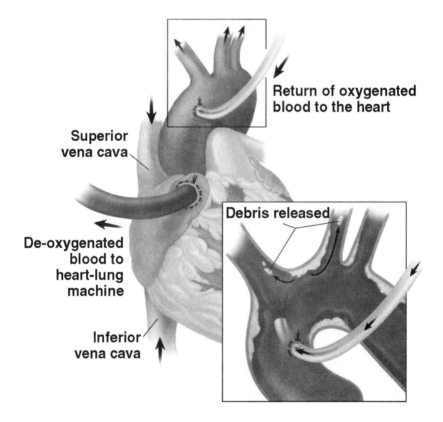

Figure 11.9. Power-spray effect of flow from the heart-lung machine. The force of blood under pressure from the heart-lung machine can dislodge plaque material to the brain or other organs.

with severe diffuse arteriosclerosis in many organs or those who have had a prior stroke. Also at risk are the very elderly, especially those over seventy-five or eighty years of age, who may face a stroke risk of 5 percent or more.

For these reasons, there is recent renewed interest in performing heart surgery without the heart-lung machine. The heart-lung machine is often referred to semicolloquially as the *pump*, so cases done without the heart-lung machine are referred to as *off-pump* cases. Of course, only coronary bypass can be performed in this way. Valve replacement and other procedures that require opening

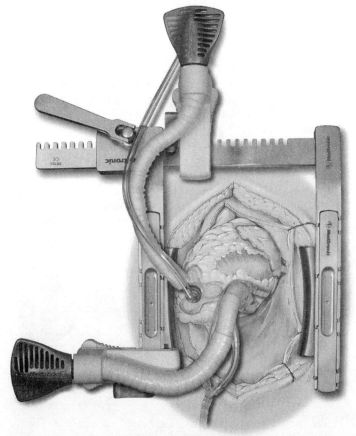

Figure 11.10. The Octopus® heart stabilizing device, a registered trademark of Medtronics, Inc. Copyright Medtronic, Inc., used with permission.

the chambers of the heart cannot be done without the heart-lung machine. This point deserves emphasis: valve surgery cannot be done without the heart-lung machine. In this sense, there is no real minimally invasive alternative for patients needing valve surgery.

Many centers now offer coronary artery bypass surgery without the heart-lung machine. Devices are available that stabilize the heart to permit cutting and delicate suturing to be done to the tiny coronary arteries.

Technical devices have been developed to keep blood out of the surgeon's way during "off-pump" coronary artery bypass. Yet, there is no doubt that surgery done this way is not as controlled as that done with the heart-lung machine, which provides a still, bloodless microsurgical field. Yet, with recent advances, off-pump coronary artery bypass is becoming more and more reliable. Patency rates, the chances that the bypasses will function, are approaching those of conventional surgery.

How should I go: Off-pump or conventional bypass surgery?

Is off-pump coronary artery bypass for you? Carefully done clinical studies are now accumulating that compare bypass done both ways, with the heart-lung machine and without. It is difficult to demonstrate any real, across-the-board advantages to avoiding use of the heart-lung machine. Patency rates, mortality rates, stroke rates, and length of hospital stay are about the same. For this reason, it is best for your surgeon to apply the technique he feels is best for you— with the heart-lung machine or without. Most surgeons have a preference.

If your vessels are small, or diffusely diseased, the operation cannot be done safely without the technical advantages afforded by the heart-lung machine. Your surgeon will explain such issues to you based on the pictures he has of your coronary arteries.

Certain select groups of patients have been shown to do better by avoiding the heart-lung machine for their bypass operations. Patients who do better with off-pump bypass are those with heavy debris in their aorta. Stroke rate is somewhat lower by virtue of avoiding the sandblasting effect of the flow from the pump and its dislodgement of debris to the brain. However, even off-pump bypass usually involves some manipulation of the aorta, so the stroke rate, although somewhat lower, is by no means zero. Similarly, patients with a prior stroke in their history (especially from disease of the carotid arteries, the big arteries in the neck that deliver blood to the brain) appear to do better by avoiding the heart-lung machine. This is thought to be because the heart-lung machine delivers nonpulsatile blood flow (a constant stream), rather than the up-and-down phasic flow that results from the native heartbeat. The phasic flow pattern of the native heart appears to pump blood more effectively through carotid arteries that harbor tight blockages.

As you can see from this description, there is no consensus even among heart surgeons about which technique is best—on-pump or off-pump—for coronary artery bypass. It is advisable for you to ask your surgeon his general preferences and his preferences in your particular case. With the informational background contained in the paragraphs you have just read, you should be prepared to understand his recommendations and to express your personal preferences.

Can my operation be done by a robot?

Robotic technology is advancing to the point at which simple bypass operations (single-bypass procedures to the artery on the front of the heart, the LAD) have been performed through small port (keyhole) incisions in the chest. Most such procedures have been done on an

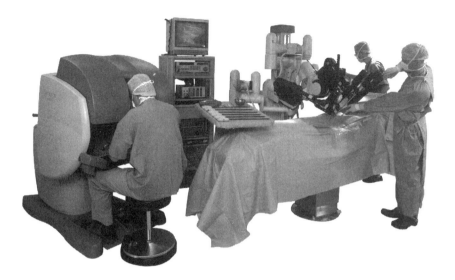

Figure 11.11. A robotic device for cardiac surgery. Copyright © 2006 Intuitive Surgical, Inc.

experimental basis in Europe. Preliminary results appear satisfactory. Clinical trials are just beginning in the United States.

In the United States, most patients with single-vessel disease would not even have surgery, rather, they would be treated by medicines or by angioplasty (see below). Eventually, the robotic technology may evolve to the point at which more complex, multivessel bypass procedures are done this way. As this book is being written, large hospitals throughout the country are purchasing robots mainly as a high-tech image-building effort. It is unlikely that you would be offered robotic coronary bypass surgery. If you are, you should recognize that this is entirely an experiment in clinical research. The authors do feel, however, that in the next two or three decades, the majority of cardiac operations may come to be done via robotic means.

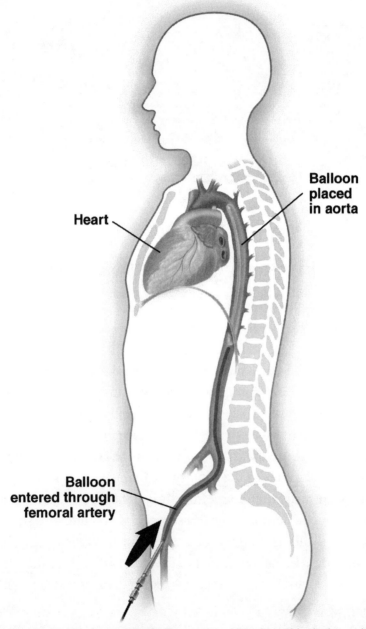

Figure 11.12. The intra-aortic balloon pump. Note how this device resides temporarily in the aorta, behind the heart, silently augmenting the heart's function.

What in the world is a "balloon" pump?

This remarkable invention has saved thousands of lives. The formal name is *intra-aortic balloon pump* or IABP, but in the hospital jargon, it is known simply as "the balloon."

This is an auxiliary pump that is the size and shape of a large sausage. It is collapsed and threaded on a pencil-sized catheter through the large artery in your groin to lie behind the heart in the main blood vessel called the *descending aorta*. By inflating and deflating in synchrony with your heart, the balloon takes a great load off your heart.

The balloon may be placed before operation, in the catheterization laboratory, to relieve your angina or stabilize your heart until surgery. The balloon may also be placed during operation if it is anticipated that your heart will need extra help.

By virtue of its technical characteristics of operation, the balloon pump not only relieves the load of pumping blood from your heart, but it also provides more nutrient blood flow to your heart (even forcing flow through blocked arteries). The synergistic sum of these two mechanisms is astoundingly powerful. At any time, a large cardiac hospital will have six to twelve patients on the balloon. This device, although remarkably effective, is not cutting-edge therapy—it has been widely used clinically for well over twenty years.

When you no longer need the balloon, it is simply withdrawn from your leg and manual pressure is applied to control the entry site.

How do I choose a heart surgeon?

Choosing your heart surgeon is not a trivial matter. In some cases, especially if you are in the process of having a heart attack or are in imminent danger of suffering one, you may not have the time to conduct a detailed search for the ideal surgeon. If your situation is not urgent—and for most patients, it is not—you should take the time to choose carefully.

Before you look for a heart surgeon, you will almost always have already seen a cardiologist; in fact, in most cases, you will have undergone a cardiac catheterization before being referred for surgery. The cardiologist who has evaluated you will likely recommend a surgeon or give you a list from which to choose. Your cardiologist's recommendations are very important. Especially if you have known him for some time, you may have confidence in his recommendations. On occasion, the cardiologist's recommendation may be based on a working relationship with the surgeon, who may not necessarily be the best person for the job in your case. It is important for you to bring other factors into consideration. Chances are that friends or family will know a surgeon who has treated others in your area. Your internist or general practitioner may be able to help in your selection. If you know a doctor in your area through other contacts or friends, you can call to see if he is comfortable with the surgeon recommended to you.

A word should be said about the published cardiac surgery statistics provided by a number of states on a yearly basis. Several states rank surgeons and hospitals on the basis of mortality rates. While there is certainly some merit in this data, it can also be very misleading. In states where such tabulations are done, surgeons and hospitals often avoid high-risk patients for the sole purpose of keeping their statistics low. That would be like if the New York Yankees only played high school baseball teams; they would likely have a perfect record. In fact, it is often the highest risk patients who need surgery the most; without surgery their outlook might be grim. Yet surgeons and hospitals that accept such patients may not rank lowest in mortality. In other words, statistical lists provided by states may be misleading if they are not "risk adjusted." Risk adjustment is not a simple process; it requires an attention to data collection and sophistication in statistical analysis that usually are beyond the resources of the collecting agencies.

Probably the most important factor in your selection of a surgeon is the feeling that you and your family get in visiting with him before surgery. (We use the word *him* because among the 2,000 cardiac surgeons in the United States, only 94 are women. We are anxious to train more women in this profession.) What is his educational background? Did he go to a good college, to a respected medical school, did he do his clinical training at a well-recognized hospital? Did he answer your questions thoroughly? Did he inspire your confidence? If the answers are yes, chances are that he should be your choice. A number of "Best Doctors" lists have been published according to specialty. These are of some merit. It is likely that the doctors whose names appear in these books and magazines are excellent. Conversely, many excellent clinical practitioners may not be well enough known outside their immediate environment to achieve such a listing; they may still give you excellent care.

Chances are that you may meet other members of your surgeon's team during your visit. Specifically, you may meet the nurse or nurses who work with the doctor in arranging surgery and communicating with families before, during, and after surgery. These are important team members, and it is helpful if you feel a positive rapport during the preoperative visit.

One more word of advice. It is your life that is at stake. If you would like to see one or more surgeons to enlist their viewpoints and recommendations, you should certainly do this. If one surgeon objects to such second or third opinions, you should avoid him. No practitioner should be so arrogant as not to be interested in the opinion of another professional or to deny you the benefit of such a consultation.

My doctor wants to put me into a research protocol. I don't want to be a "guinea pig." Is there any benefit to me? How should I reply?

At academic institutions, it is quite possible that you could be asked if you wish to participate in a cardiac research protocol of some kind intended for patients with your particular disease pattern. Please be assured of the following. No protocol is approved without the intense scrutiny of the hospital's investigational review board. This board is composed of dispassionate individuals—different individuals from your potential research team, from many different callings, not only doctors but also students, clergy, lawyers, ethicists, and statisticians. Their sole purpose is to safeguard the rights and well-being of potential research subjects. In many cases, the Food and Drug Administration will also have approved the experimental treatment, giving you another layer of protection.

Remember also that you have no obligation to participate in the research study. Your medical team must provide you excellent care whether or not you decide to participate.

In some cases, the experimental treatment—for example, a new drug, new procedure, or new device—may actually be of benefit to you. In other cases, the potential benefit may not be for you but rather for the future of humankind.

For many, if not most, research studies, patients will be randomized—that is, some will be in the "treatment" group and others in the "placebo" group. The treatment group receives an active drug, while the placebo group receives a nonactive replica (usually a sugar pill). Having the patients randomized allows us to evaluate much more accurately whether the experimental therapy is actually effective.

In some cases, investigators can be overzealous in pursuing your participation in a research study. One of your authors required an emergency procedure in a foreign country where he was serving as a visiting professor. He was alone, without friends or family, and some five thousand miles away from the United States. His treating physicians would not take no for an answer, and even as he was being wheeled in to the procedure room, doctor after doctor arrived with a permission form in hand, waving a pen for signature. Your author, under these circumstances, steadfastly refused to give permission, and was rendered routine therapy only.

You should follow your conscience when asked about a research protocol. If you are at an institution you know well, among caregivers whom you trust, and you have family and friends with whom to discuss the pros and cons, you may wish to give permission to be included in a scientific study. It is through the generous participation of patients who choose to participate in research projects after detailed informed consent that medical progress is made. It is organized research protocols that provide definitive answers to important questions in medicine.

Chapter
12
SURGICAL PROCEDURES

CORONARY ARTERY BYPASS GRAFTING

Who needs a bypass operation?

There are several indications for the coronary artery bypass operation. *Indication* is the medical term for the appropriate scenario in which a certain type of therapy should be applied.

The first set of indications for the bypass operation has to do with functional criteria; that is, with issues of how you are getting along, or coping, with your coronary artery disease. If you have no angina, you may not need a bypass operation. Or if you have a stable, tolerable pattern of angina, you may not need a bypass operation. If, however, your angina is disabling to the point that your quality of life is adversely affected or you cannot carry out the activities of daily life—like work, recreation, or family life—a bypass operation may be appropriate for you. A bypass operation is also appropriate for patients who have an unstable anginal pattern, one that is increasing in frequency or severity.

Also, if you are in the hospital with a heart attack in progress or the threat of a heart attack, a bypass operation may be important to keep these events controlled by supplying more blood flow to the threatened areas of heart muscle.

The second set of indications for the bypass operation has to do with anatomic criteria, that is, issues of extent and severity of the actual blockages. If you have severe disease of the most important artery of the heart, the left main coronary artery, you need surgery. Likewise, if you have disease of all three arteries of the heart and you have had significant damage to your heart from a prior heart attack, you need bypass surgery. If you have less disease, say, of only one or two arteries, and you feel well and get along, you may not need a bypass operation.

God overdesigned our coronary arteries, like everything else in our bodies. The amount of blood flow through your vessel is not impaired until a blockage equals or exceeds 60 to 75 percent. Thus, when we talk about significant blockages in one, two, or three arteries, we mean only blockages exceeding those percentages.

Your doctor may bring other factors to bear on the decision for bypass surgery. For example, if you did very poorly on your exercise test, with a drop in blood pressure, abnormal heartbeats, severe EKG changes, or abnormalities on imaging suggesting a large amount of heart muscle at risk, a bypass operation may be very important for you. Similarly, if these worrisome changes were brought on early via exercise, that is also concerning and suggests bypass surgery may be important for you.

The decision for or against bypass may at times be simple and at other times more complex. You need to discuss this issue carefully with your cardiologist and your heart surgeon.

What materials will you use for my grafts?

There are two widely used conduits for construction of bypass grafts.

The original and classic conduit is the vein from your leg, which we call the *greater saphenous vein*. Figure 12.1 shows the course of this vein.

Table 12.1. Indications for Coronary Bypass Surgery.

Functional indications	**Anatomic indications**
1. Threatened heart attack	1. Left main lesion
2. Incapacitating angina	2. Three-vessel disease, with
3. Unstable anginal pattern	prior heart attack

Worrisome findings on stress testing
1. Trouble early in test
2. Drop in blood pressure
3. Major EKG changes
4. Images show large area at risk

This vein is located on the inside of your thigh and lower leg. If you find the bump on the inner side of your ankle, what we call the *medial malleolus*, you may be able to see the vein just in front of that bump. If you stand up, the vein will fill with blood. You may see the bluish streak representing the blood in this vein. You may be able to feel the vein full of blood when you stand or sit with your

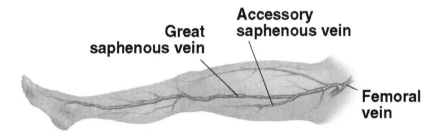

Figure 12.1. The course of the greater saphenous vein. This is a superficial venous system, located just under the skin. We make a shallow incision right over the course of this vein to harvest it for use. This vein is different from the femoral vein, also shown, the important deep system that drains the leg. The large-volume femoral vein system is unaffected by harvesting of the greater saphenous vein; the deep system will continue to drain blood from your leg.

feet on the floor. This vein is only the superficial vein of your leg, carrying only a small amount of the total blood flow returning from your leg to your body. (Remember, veins carry blood back to the heart from other organs. Arteries carry blood from the heart to other organs. The bypass operation does not use any arteries from your leg.) The deep vein from your leg carries 95 percent of the blood flow. After we use the superficial vein for your bypass operation, the deep vein will take on the small extra burden.

The other common conduit is the internal mammary artery. This has become very popular since 1983. This is the artery that runs on the inner aspect of your breastbone, just to either side. You have two of them. Both men and women have them. These arteries supply blood to the rib cage, the breastbone, and the breasts, for which the artery is named. This is a great conduit for bypass grafts, with exceptional long-term results, as discussed below.

How is the bypass procedure actually performed?

Figures 12.2a and 12.2b illustrate the bypass operation schematically, and figures 12.3a–k show actual operating room photographs of the operation, some taken with extreme magnification.

Usually, the connections of the conduits to the coronary arteries, which we call the *distal anastomoses*, are constructed first. *Distal* means "farther along an anatomic structure" and *anastomoses* means "hookup." The tiny artery is incised with a blade and then the incision is extended with a scissors. The length of the opening is about five millimeters and the width is about one to two millimeters. The conduit and the artery are attached by about a dozen and a half stitches taken with a single running suture. The suture is pulled up to parachute the conduit down onto the artery. Note that the conduit is sewn to an opening made in the side of the coronary artery. The artery is not cut in half. The diseased artery is not

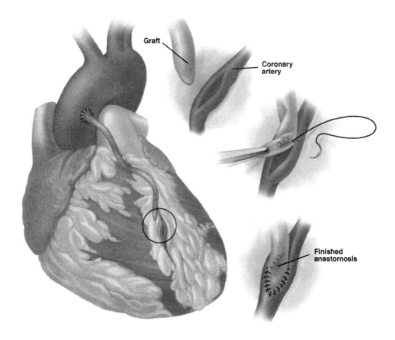

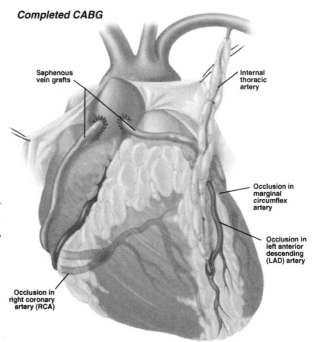

Completed CABG

Figures 12.2a and 12.2b. The coronary bypass operation, illustrated. Part a shows how we open the coronary artery and do the hookup with a vein. Part b shows the completed operation. Note that this represents a "triple" bypass, with two vein grafts and one mammary graft, all of which are shown.

Part A

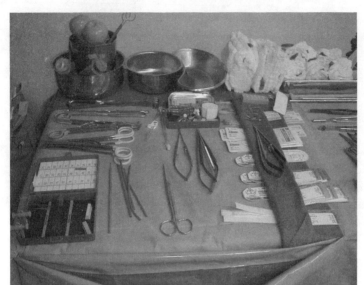

Part B

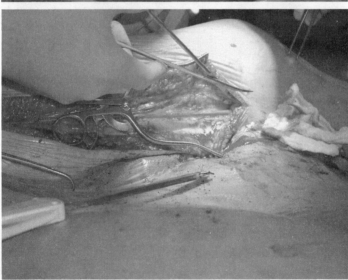

Figures 12.3a–k. The coronary bypass operation, actual operative photographs. Part a shows the table of fine instruments used for the delicate suturing of the coronary vessels. Part b shows the vein being harvested from the thigh. In this figure, the head of the patient is to your left and the foot is to your right. You can see the knee just above the surgeon's scissors. Part c shows the vein harvested and being prepared on the back table. Part d shows the heart exposed for surgery. You are looking down from the head of the table. Part e shows the tubings from the

heart-lung machine being placed into the heart chambers. Part f shows the important LAD artery being incised for hookup. Part g shows a close-up of this incision. The LAD is running left to right. Part h shows an extreme close-up of the suturing process. Note that several stitches have been taken between the open coronary artery below and the mammary artery above. The needle is being passed outside-in through the wall of the mammary artery. Remember that the mammary artery is only 1.5 millimeters in diameter (like the lead in a pencil). The suture material itself is just visible to the naked eye. Part i shows the mammary artery being "parachuted" down into place onto the coronary artery, after a number of sutures have been placed. Part j shows the mammary artery now in place. You can see that additional sutures need to be placed to complete the hookup. Part k shows the completed anastomosis (blood vessel hookup). The mammary artery is now connected to the LAD coronary artery. The LAD can be seen as the thin white structure that runs toward the lower righthand corner of the photograph.

Part C

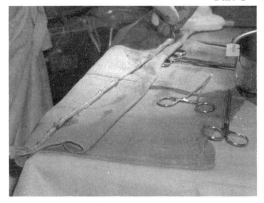

Part D

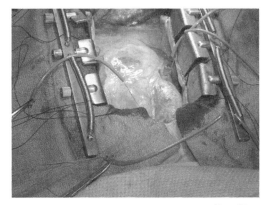

Part E

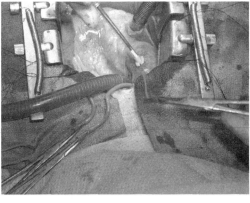

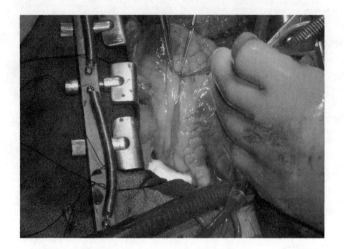

Part F

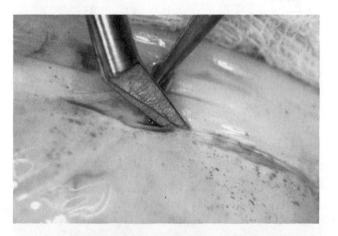

Part G

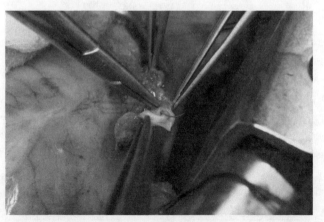

Part H

Part I

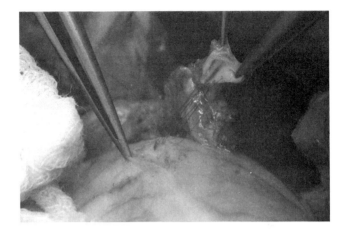

Part J

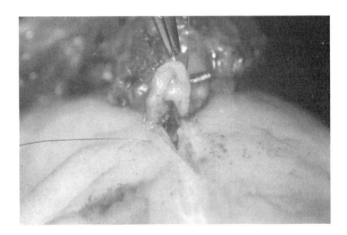

Part K

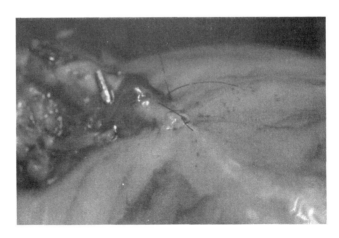

removed. This would be impossible to do, and unnecessary as well. The hookup is done beyond the last blockage, thus "bypassing" the blockage and providing free blood flow to the heart muscle.

After the hookup to the coronary artery is done, the vein is connected to the aorta, or the main artery of the body, so that the vein may receive blood flow to carry to the heart. This is called the *proximal*, or upper anastomoses, because it is located upstream to the heart. This hookup is done by punching a five-millimeter hole in the aorta and again suturing with a running stitch taken many times through both structures. The end of the vein is sewn to a hole in the side of the aorta.

If the bypass is done with the mammary artery, no proximal anastomosis is necessary, as nature has already done that. The mammary artery comes already attached to a great source of inflow, the subclavian artery, the main artery to your arm.

How long will the bypass last?

It is helpful to consider the specific fate of the individual bypasses constructed as part of a coronary artery bypass operation.[1] The major conduits used to construct the bypass are the leg veins and the mammary artery. These will be considered in turn.

First of all, not all individual bypass grafts constructed at operation will function effectively. About 95 percent of the bypasses will "take"—that is, carry blood and remain open. This is the percentage that are functioning at one month after the operation. This percentage is about the same for all conduits; that is, for both vein grafts and for the mammary artery.

It is not surprising that the early function rate is not 100 percent. Few things are 100 percent in life. When you think of all the factors that must play themselves out just right for an individual bypass graft to function, it's actually surprising that so many vein grafts do function, as clinical research has shown to be true. For the graft to "take," many, many factors must play themselves out perfectly. The target artery must have a soft area where the bypass may be placed. The target area must irrigate a sufficient area of heart muscle for there to be a relatively large, high-velocity flow of blood through the bypass. The vein or other conduit must be of good quality and must tolerate the mechanical trauma of being harvested and stored (albeit briefly) until use. All of the eighteen or twenty sutures must be perfectly placed, so none encroaches on the opening, or *lumen*, through which blood flow passes. This is no mean feat, as all these sutures are placed into an artery that is one to two millimeters in diameter, or about the thickness of the lead in a number 2 pencil. Imagine placing so many fine sutures around the perimeter of such a small structure. Also, no clots must form at the slightly irritated zones where the stitches cross the wall of the artery or vein. Similar events must occur at the end where the vein is attached to the aorta at its upper, or *proximal* end. Furthermore, the length and lie of the graft, after both ends are attached, must be perfect and smooth, without kinking or tension or excess length. The body must avoid forming excess swelling at the sites of connection of blood vessels. Later on, the body must avoid depositing excess scar tissue at the sites of hookup of blood vessels. As you may know, a scar in the skin can become heaped up and thick. If the same happens internally at the site where the vein is attached to the coronary artery, a narrowing and possible closure of the bypass graft will occur. Thus, the excellent 95 percent patency rate of bypass grafts is a miracle of sorts, which to this day fascinates your authors, despite their own application of this operation in thousands upon thousands of patients.

Now, let's move on in time to the ten-year point. Are the bypasses still open? Well, for the vein grafts, about 40 percent will have closed and 60 percent will still be open. Why will some have closed? The reason is recurrent arteriosclerosis. More disease may attack your vein graft or the artery to which it attaches, leading to closure. Not all bypasses are so affected. In fact, even within the same single patient, some vein grafts may become diseased while others remain pristine. We do not understand the reasons for such differences.

At the ten-year point, however, the situation is much different for the mammary graft. Nearly the same 95 percent that were open at one month are still open at ten years. The mammary artery is essentially immune to arteriosclerosis. We do not know why this is true, but we are glad that it is so. The favorable behavior of the mammary artery used as a bypass graft is so impressive that some surgeons have speculated that God put it on the inside of the chest wall so that it could be used for this very purpose.

The good news does not end there. Let's go on to fifteen and twenty years after your bypass. Believe it or not, the same 95 percent of mammary grafts that were patent and functioning at one month and at ten years are still open and pumping at fifteen and twenty years. Those mammary grafts just keep on pumping. They are almost lifelong, even if disease in your original coronary arteries progresses.

Figure 12.4 shows the percentage of both kinds of grafts still functioning at various times after the performance of the bypass operation. The superiority of the mammary bypass operation is clearly evident.

I have heard that my vein can be harvested without an incision. Is this feasible?

In recent years, multiple commercial systems have been developed that permit the saphenous vein to be harvested with only two small incisions used for introduction of a harvesting "scope." One pop-

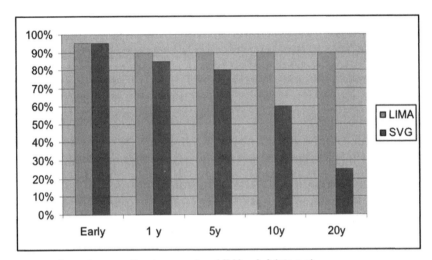

Long-term graft patency rates. LIMA = left internal
mammary graft. SVG = saphenous vein graft.

Figure 12.4. Long-term graft patency rates.

ular harvesting system is called the Vaso-View system. Such noninvasive harvesting produces benefits in terms of pain, mobility,
and wound healing in the leg. This method of harvesting is very
popular with patients. In the best of circumstances, the patient is
hardly aware that any work has been done on his leg.

There are some pertinent negatives to this type of harvest. This
technique usually yields adequate vein area for two bypasses. If
you need more than two vein grafts, chances are that your incision
will be extended conventionally, with a scalpel and an incision.

The biological behavior of veins harvested conventionally is
well known. We know that these grafts have a 94 percent patency
rate, or likelihood of functioning well and remaining open, in the
short term. Comparable studies on Vaso-View–harvested veins are
simply not available. There are reasons to postulate that the trauma
to the vein is greater with a Vaso-View harvest, and that patency
rates could be adversely affected. Any detriment in patency cannot

be great, however, as such has not been clinically apparent in the many thousands of cases done this way. But detailed studies, with angiography to confirm patency, are, frankly, lacking.

There are many instances in medicine where it has taken decades to realize the wisdom or folly of new techniques.

Your authors' advice regarding the noninvasive harvesting of vein for the bypass operation is that it is a reasonable technique, producing increased patient comfort and satisfaction, but that the jury is still out on the long-term consequences.

What about the grafts taken from the arm?

The radial artery is the artery that runs along the thumb side of your forearm. Although this is an artery, not a vein, it can usually be taken safely for use on your heart because it has a counterpart on the other side of the forearm. It is the counterpart that will supply your hand with blood if you have a radial artery graft.

Many surgeons believe that the radial artery makes a good bypass graft for the heart because nature made it an artery, unlike the veins from your leg. In fact, it is hard to prove that the radial artery performs any better than vein grafts. The radial artery can be very finicky, and some early problems with spasm or closure are occasionally seen. Also, unlike the mammary graft, which is left attached to the subclavian artery, the radial artery, because it is removed entirely from your arm, requires a proximal anastomosis (or hookup) to your aorta. This makes it a less natural arrangement than a mammary bypass.

The bypass operation is an art. Your surgeon will have his own preferences concerning conduits. He will quite likely discuss conduit choices with you.

What about the grafts taken from the belly?

In certain cases, we actually borrow one of the four arteries that provide blood supply to your stomach to use on your heart. The stomach has abundant blood supply and will not miss the "borrowed" artery. This artery is called the gastroepiploic artery. It is not used as frequently as other conduits because it is a bit awkward to harvest and can be quite small at certain levels. It can be a wonderful conduit for bypass graft, however, with excellent long-term patency. It does not require a proximal anastomosis, as it comes already attached to the aorta in your abdomen. Only the free end is swung over to your heart.

If the mammary artery bypass is so wonderful, why will I only have one mammary-based bypass? Don't I have two mammary arteries inside my chest, after all, a left one and a right one?

This is a very good question. Believe it or not, the right mammary does not perform as well as the left as a conduit for the bypass operation. Why in the world would this be? Didn't Nature make the two mammary arteries equal? Indeed, she did, but it is the left mammary that is an easy reach to the most important artery on your heart, the left anterior descending, or LAD. Part of the reason that the left mammary bypass does so well is that it is placed onto the LAD, which keeps a large volume of blood flowing at all times.

The right mammary does not reach as well to important targets, as the heart is located a bit more to the left side of the chest. Because it is a more difficult reach, the right mammary artery is not used as frequently as the left in the coronary artery bypass operation. Also, because the right mammary graft is accustomed to secondary arteries, smaller and with less flow, its results are not as strikingly superb.

If the patient is young, say, sixty-five or less, we are inclined to find some way to use both mammary arteries, in the hopes of providing a very durable result from the bypass operation.

Are there any drawbacks to using both the right and left mammary arteries in the bypass operation? Yes. The breastbone will have less blood flow for healing if both arteries are used. If you are a diabetic, you can expect a higher incidence of infection of the breast incision after the operation, from a 2 percent to a 4 percent likelihood. As long as you understand this, your surgeon may still choose this option, for the benefits of two arterial grafts in your long-term future.

Can the bypass procedure be done a second time?

Yes, the bypass can be done a second time, if necessary. It is more difficult and dangerous the second time, for many reasons. You will be older. Your cardiac structures will be stuck together inside—what we call adhesions—because of the irritation to internal membranes from the first operation. The selection for location of bypass on your coronary arteries will be "second choice," so to speak. Also, there are many other technical complicating features. But experienced medical centers offer second-time operations with confidence and good expectations.

The operation is sometimes performed a third time, if necessary, and, rarely, a fourth. In one case, your authors performed a sixth-time coronary artery bypass operation. The benefit becomes more limited with these multiple performances, and the dangers mount swiftly with the number of operations.

How many arteries are there on the heart?

Each of us is born with three major arteries that run on the surface of the heart and provide the heart muscle with blood. These are one to three millimeters in diameter, or from about the size of pencil lead to the size of the refill in your ballpoint pen. A patient can have *single-vessel* disease, *double-vessel* disease, or *triple-vessel* disease. It is essential to recognize that each of these main arteries divides into literally innumerable smaller tributaries, like the branches of a tree. One can count any number of arteries. We customarily count only the three major branches and their major tributaries.

You will hear your cardiologist or surgeon use the names of the blocked arteries or the ones bypassed. You can review the anatomy of the coronary arteries in chapter 1, figure 1.2.

The left coronary arises as what we call the *left main* coronary artery. This in turn divides into the left anterior descending coronary artery and the circumflex coronary artery. The left anterior coronary artery (or LAD) is the single most important artery of your heart, supplying 40 percent of your heart's total blood flow. This one is called the "widow maker," in recognition of the devastating impact of a sudden occlusion of this vital tributary. This left anterior descending coronary artery courses down the very front of your heart. The circumflex runs around the left side of your heart to supply blood to the side, or lateral wall, of your heart.

The right coronary artery arises separately and runs along the right side of the heart to supply the bottom, or "inferior wall" of the heart.

You will also come across the names of the branches of the coronary arteries. The branches of the left anterior descending coronary artery are called *diagonals* when they run to the side of the main vessel, or *septals* when they course directly deep into the heart muscle. The branches of the circumflex coronary artery are called the *marginals*. The main branch of the right coronary artery is the posterior descending coronary artery, or PDA. You can use the diagram in figure 1.2 to locate the arteries that your doctors discuss with you. This diagram will also serve to indicate what regions of your heart are irrigated by the different arteries your doctors will describe.

The pain related to blockages in the different arteries is felt in the center of the chest. The right coronary artery doesn't cause pain on the right, nor does the left coronary artery cause pain on the left. The body cannot discriminate between insufficient blood flow caused by the different arteries.

My friend had six bypasses; why can't I have the same?

You may not need that many grafts. There is a saying among heart surgeons, promulgated by one of our colleagues, Dr. Gary Kopf, that no one ever died with three good bypass grafts. There is a lot of wisdom in that saying. More is not necessarily better. More bypasses means more time on the heart-lung machine, and more cross-clamp time, both of which may be dangerous to your health or your life. Some smaller arteries may not sustain the grafts, so the extra work is wasted.

In general, most surgeons would graft each artery that is blocked more than 60 percent and that is larger than 1.5 millimeters in diameter. This may make for one graft in one patient or five or six in another. Three is the most common number of bypasses performed on a single patient.

Will my angina go away after my bypass?

About three-fourths of patients will have complete relief of their angina. Many of the remainder will gain substantial relief in terms of frequency or severity of angina. Some few patients do not benefit, for a variety of reasons. Their bypasses may not all function well, or even a small artery, not big enough to bypass, may cause severe angina. In general, however, the bypass operation is very effective in relieving symptoms of angina.

It is worthwhile to note that up to 15 percent of patients may require some angioplasty "touch-up work" in the first year after bypass surgery.

How will I know if my bypasses are working?

If you are feeling well, without chest pain or significant shortness of breath with exertion, it is likely that your bypasses are working fine. How you feel is the single most important and overriding factor in the assessment of your bypass operation.

Your cardiologist may also do a stress test periodically to assess your heart's response to exercise.

Can you treat me with a laser instead of a bypass?

Lasers have been used in two different ways in heart care. Some ten years ago, it was hoped that a fine laser beam could be used to bore a precise, atraumatic opening through coronary artery blockages. Considerable laboratory and clinical work was done on this technique. It did not prove that helpful, and the laser is not used frequently in the present day to open blocked arteries.

The other way that the laser has been used is for a technique called *transmyocardial laser revascularization* or TMR. This tech-

nique was developed in the hope of helping patients without adequate target arteries for a conventional bypass operation. Without
an adequate area of soft artery on which to "touch down," a bypass
with a mammary artery or a saphenous vein cannot be performed.
Many patients suffer from such lack of suitable target arteries. We
say that these patients have *diffuse* disease, which means that
instead of having localized blockages at the start of the arteries, the
arteries are blocked up and down throughout their length.

Diffuse disease is most common in patients with long-standing
diabetes or severe hyperlipidemia.

The TMR technique takes a different approach. This technique
drills holes right through the heart muscle, from the outside to the
inside. It was originally hoped that these channels would stay open
and carry blood directly from the chambers of the heart to irrigate
the heart muscle. This technique of heart irrigation actually occurs
in nature—in reptiles and alligators.

It has now been shown that the channels do not, in fact, remain
open. Yet the procedure is effective in reducing or eliminating
anginal pain in patients with no other options. This TMR procedure
is used occasionally in current clinical practice.

Studies to see if TMR actually increases blood flow to the heart
muscle have yielded equivocal results. It may be that TMR does
indeed produce a modest improvement in blood flow—possibly by
producing a scar in the heart muscle, which carries blood vessels
with it. Alternatively, it may be that the laser simply destroys some
columns of cardiac muscle, in essence *denervating* the heart—
destroying the nerve fibers responsible for sensing anginal pain in
that region.

Our bottom line advice on the laser procedure of TMR is that it
may be appropriate in a small number of angina patients. However,
if you are a candidate for a conventional coronary artery bypass
procedure, that is a much better alternative.

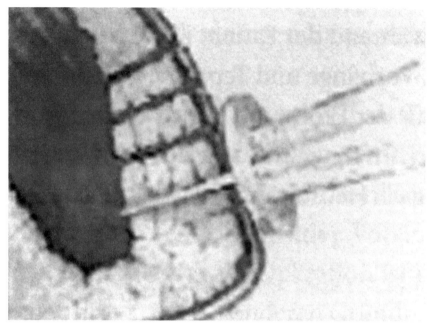

Figure 12.5. The transmyocardial laser procedure, courtesy of Edwards Lifesciences, Irvine, California.

After my bypass operation, can I eat anything I want or do I still need to watch my cholesterol?

Your bypass operation is just plumbing, albeit very delicate plumbing. The coronary artery bypass has absolutely no effect on the chemistry of your body that caused the deposits to develop in the first place. Your cholesterol and other lipids will resume their prior levels when your diet stabilizes after surgery. Controlling your cholesterol and other risk factors will be just as important after your operation. Without controlling your risk factors, you may not gain as much benefit from your new bypasses. By controlling these risk factors, you will ensure that your bypasses continue to function as long as possible.

Far and away the most significant risk factor for you to control after coronary bypass surgery is cigarette smoking. *If you smoke, your bypasses will close.* It is that plain and that simple. You must never smoke another cigarette after your bypass operation. You will have been smoke-free for all the days that you were in the hospital. Take this opportunity to continue your smoke-free state, and you will do your bypasses and your overall health a big favor. The benefits to your family will be great; you will help ensure that you will be around to enjoy their company for the longest possible time.

It may be wise for the family to carry out some supportive maneuvers regarding smoking cessation while the patient is in the hospital. The family can clean the home environment, dry-clean the drapes, steam-clean the rugs, and so on to remove the smell of smoke from the house. The car interior can be cleaned too. We want the patient to never, ever have another cigarette after returning home.

Is the coronary bypass operation a proven form of treatment?

Not only is the coronary artery bypass procedure a proven form of treatment, but some authorities, including your authors, feel it ranks as *one of the most proven modalities of treatment in the history of humankind.* The procedure of coronary artery bypass surgery has been performed since the mid-1960s. For many years now, more than four hundred thousand such operations have been performed yearly in the United States alone. The procedure has been tested "every which way but sideways." The bypass procedure has been tested in many carefully designed multicenter randomized clinical trials, the most stringent mechanisms for evaluating any treatment modalities. Time after time, the evaluations have demonstrated that the procedure works, and works very well. It has been shown that: (1) Bypass surgery is safe. (2) The individual bypass grafts actually work. (3) Patients' symptoms (usually angina) are relieved by the bypass operation. (4) Patients' lives are prolonged by the operation. (5) The bypass operation can restore some of the pumping strength of the heart that has been lost over years of heart disease. And (6) benefits of the coronary artery bypass operation are very durable.

Benefits of Coronary Artery Bypass Graft (CABG)

1. Safe
2. Effective
3. Relieves angina
4. Prolongs life
5. Restores pumping strength
6. Benefits are durable

Another testimony to the effectiveness of the coronary bypass operation is that results of most if not all of the formal trials have been interpreted in whole or in large part not by surgeons but by cardiologists. This should eliminate most fears of undue bias, as cardiologists do not perform coronary bypass procedures, and thus have no reason to wish to see its benefits exaggerated. In fact, cardiologists have multiple conflicting technologies that they themselves offer, so their strong support of the coronary artery bypass operation speaks volumes.

VALVE REPLACEMENT

A common joke among medical practitioners is that cardiac surgeons only do three operations: coronary bypass, mitral valve replacement, and aortic valve replacement. While this is an exaggeration, valve surgery is a very important part of what we do. Valve disease, from congenital malformations, wear and tear of age, or infection, is quite common. In this section, we address your questions on valve surgery.

What are the kinds of replacement valves?

There are two general types of artificial heart valves: animal (or tissue) valves and mechanical valves. Each type has specific advantages and potential liabilities. These valves are shown in the figure below.

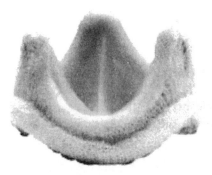 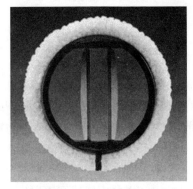

Figures 12.6 left and 12.6 right. Replacement heart valves. On the left is an animal valve (Edwards Bovine Pericardial Valve) and on the right is a mechanical valve (St. Jude Valve), courtesy of the manufacturers.

Animal valves generally are made from tissues from pigs (called porcine valves) or cows (bovine valves).

The pig valves are generally removed directly from animals grown specifically for this purpose, then mounted on delicate hardware that supports the valve and incorporates a sewing ring to facilitate securing to the patient's heart. These valves are natural, in the sense that they functioned in the animal from which they were removed.

In the case of valves from cows, the tissue is actually removed from the cow's pericardium, the strong material that makes up the sac that surrounds every mammal's heart. This raw material, like a thick plastic wrap in consistency, is precisely and delicately fashioned into humanmade leaflets. Three of these leaflets are incorporated to make up a valve. The finished product incorporates a cloth sewing ring. The valves come prepared, packed in preservative, and ready for implantation directly off the shelf.

Occasionally, we may use a valve taken from an expired human being. These are called *homograft* valves. Their function and longevity are comparable to those of animal valves.

The mechanical valves are completely man made. They are made from a material called *pyrolite carbon*, which is the same substance from which artificial diamonds are made. This material is very hard and smooth, so it does not attract blood clots. Several manufacturers make valves from this material under different product names. These valves also incorporate a cloth sewing ring.

All the valve types come in a variety of sizes, and a complete range of sizes is in stock in the operating room. The process is similar to shoe sizing. Every individual has a different size annulus (see below) into which the valve needs to be placed. A sizing instrument is placed into the site in the heart where the new valve will fit in order to measure the size needed. A valve in the appropriate size is taken from the shelf for your use.

How do you attach the valve to my heart?

The first step in replacing your valve is to remove the old, diseased valve. It is excised by scissors or blade. This leaves a soft but strong fibrous ring, called the *annulus*. It is to this annulus that the new valve is sewn. A series of sutures are placed through the annulus, usually about twelve to twenty, and then passed through the cloth ring of the artificial valve. When these sutures are tied, the valve "parachutes" into place within the annulus of your heart. A watertight, secure attachment results. This process is shown in the figure below. The process is quite similar in both the mitral and aortic positions.

In time, your body will reinforce this attachment by growing tissue into the interstices in the cloth of the sewing ring of the valve. However, the secure attachment of your valve will always be dependent on the placement sutures. The material of these sutures, reassuringly, is essentially lifelong. Even decades later, the sutures appear to be in the same condition as the day they went in.

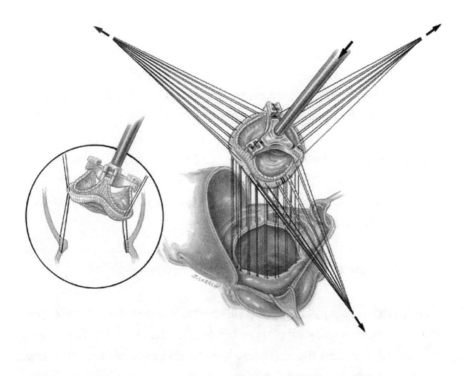

Figure 12.7. Implantation of an artificial heart valve, courtesy of Edwards Life-sciences, Irvine, California.

Can the valve be rejected?

The valve you receive, whether an animal valve or a mechanical valve, cannot be rejected because it is not alive. Transplanted organs such as hearts, livers, or kidneys can all be rejected by your body because they are alive and performing active, vital functions. In contradistinction, your heart valve, while very important, is neither alive nor performing active functions. It functions passively, opening or closing as your heart muscle propels blood forward. It is easy to understand that the mechanical valve, made of artificial, humanmade materials, is not living. However, even the animal valves are treated in such a way that living cells are removed and only the scaffold of collagen, a basic structural building block of the body, remains. The valve is not renewed by your body, unlike all your own tissues and organs, which are "rebuilt" regularly by your body's inherent renewal mechanisms. So you need not have any concern regarding rejection of your valve.

In some cases, valves are taken from dead human beings and frozen for later use as replacement valves. There is little advantage of human valves over animal valves. Even human valves "recycled" in this way are not alive and wear out in about the same length of time as animal valves.

Your new valve can, however, become infected, and that can be very serious. Because it is an artificial part, it cannot clear bacteria from its surfaces the way your own tissues can. We teach our students that the interstices in the cloth of the sewing ring provide an environment where bacterial organisms can take hold and thrive. We use the analogy that these small crevices can serve as a "luxury hotel" for bacteria, while the surrounding blood provides "room service," with all the nutrients that the bacteria require to proliferate.

However, infection is very rare with new valves. Your authors cannot recall the last time that such an event occurred with their patients. These events usually reflect some type of contamination during the surgical procedure to place the new valve or some infectious event soon afterward that forced bacteria into the bloodstream. You will be given antibiotics preventatively (*prophylactically*, is the medical term) around the time of your operation to provide extra protection from such events. The likelihood of an early infection of your valve is less than 1 percent.

The only circumstance in which such infections are common occurs when the valve replacement is being performed specifically to treat a native valve that is already infected. This is called *endocarditis*, again from the Greek, meaning infection of the inside of the heart. In such a circumstance, you will be given antibiotics for weeks to discourage any stray remaining bacteria from seeding in your clean, new valve. Nonetheless, infection does recur with some regularity in such cases, and treatment can be difficult or unfruitful, with serious or lethal consequences.

What type of valve will I need?

The two types of valves—animal and mechanical—have their own benefits and liabilities, as indicated in table 12.3.

Animal valves have the wonderful advantage of being "blood-friendly" because they are biological material; for this reason, they do not promote clotting and thus do not require blood thinners. This is a very important plus for these valves. However, the great disadvantage of animal valves is that they wear out in due course. Again, this is due to their not being alive and not being replenished or restored by your body. The collagen in the valves is what gives them their structure. It can only bend, to open and close, so many times. We explain this to our students using an expired credit card as an analogy. Many users tear up the card to avoid its unauthorized use. Those of you who have tried this, however, know that it has to be flexed and unflexed many, many times before it breaks. It is the same with the collagen in your animal valve; this can take millions upon millions of heartbeats, but, eventually, it gives way.

Table 12.3. Two Types of Valves.

	Animal valves	*Mechanical valves*
Blood thinners required?	No	Yes
Durable?	No	Yes
Ideal for...	Older patients	Younger patients
Inappropriate for...	Younger patients	Patients with bleeding problems

Animal valves can be expected to last over a decade. In some cases, they can last fifteen or even twenty years. There is some evidence that the newest pericardial valves (cow tissue) last longer than any prior animal valves ever developed.

One interesting fact is that animal valves last a long time in older patients and a much shorter time in young people. We do not know the reason for this. In an adolescent or young adult, for example, an animal valve may break down even within the first five years.

Mechanical valves, by virtue of not being biologic in origin and composition, are not as friendly to the blood and tend to attract and promote microscopic blood clots.[2] For this reason, lifelong administration of blood thinners is generally recommended for patients with mechanical heart valves. (See the section titled "What is Coumadin?" in chapter 9.) The great advantage of mechanical valves is their durability. One type of valve (the so called St. Jude Valve) has been in use for thirty years and has not yet worn out. Over one million patients have received this valve. Structural failures of any kind have been almost unheard of. What will happen after thirty years, medical science cannot say, but three decades is a very, very long time in medical care, especially where the heart is involved.

Regarding the need for blood thinners, it is important to point out that patients who receive animal valves may require blood thinners for other reasons besides the valve itself. This is, in fact, quite common. Some surgeons use blood thinners for a brief period of time even after placing biological valves. In patients with valvular heart disease, an irregular rhythm of the upper chambers of the heart, called *atrial fibrillation*, is common (see the section titled "What causes atrial fibrillation?" in chapter 3). This irregular rhythm requires blood thinners, so that clots do not form in the irregularly contracting chambers of the heart. This situation can negate the advantage of animal valves vis-à-vis blood thinners.

What is this "Ross operation" I keep hearing about? Is that what I need?

This question has to do with options for aortic valve replacement. An operation is available that "borrows" your own pulmonic valve, transferring it into position to replace your aortic valve. This is called the Ross operation, after its inventive creator, British heart surgeon Sir Donald Ross. Of course, the "borrowed" pulmonic valve must be replaced by something, usually by a valve from a dead person.

The idea here is to avoid Coumadin. That is the main advantage of the Ross operation. The other underlying principle is that the pulmonic valve is less important than the aortic valve.

If you are young (less than fifty), very active physically (performing activities for which Coumadin may be risky), or if you are a young woman of childbearing age, you may want to consider a Ross operation.

If you need Coumadin for other reasons, there is probably no advantage to having a Ross operation. If you have what we call *connective tissue disease*, like Marfan syndrome, your pulmonic valve may also be weak, and you should not have a Ross procedure.

The Ross operation is a much bigger procedure than a standard aortic valve replacement, with a commensurately higher operative risk. Also, chances are that it will not last a lifetime, as either the aortic or pulmonic valve may require further surgery in the long-term future.

The Ross procedure is appropriate for only a minority of patients undergoing aortic valve replacement. If you are interested, you should discuss this carefully with your surgeon. He will have vital insights and recommendations to share with you.

Can I have a "minimally invasive" valve replacement without the heart-lung machine?

Your heart valves are located *inside* your heart. For this reason, there is no way to replace them without opening your heart. The heart must be stopped to be opened. For the heart to be stopped, you must be placed on the heart-lung machine.

The coronary bypass operation, however, can indeed be performed without the heart-lung machine, because the coronary arteries are located *on the surface* of the heart, rather than inside.

For this reason, the term *minimally invasive* valve replacement is of limited significance. Usually, this term is used to refer to some alternate incision other than a median sternotomy (see chapter 1).

Be aware, however, that since the heart-lung machine *must* be used for a valve replacement, it is inherently a maximally invasive operation.

Can't you pass the valve into my heart with a catheter, without an operation?

In the animal laboratory, incipient forays into delivering replacement valves by catheter, without an incision, are being made. Some success has been achieved. These investigational procedures have been performed to replace perfectly normal valves. These normal valves are not removed; the catheter-delivered valve is placed within the normal native valve. Initial clinical trials in patients too ill for conventional valve surgery are beginning. It is too early to know if this will prove a viable treatment modality, even in highly selected cases.

It is difficult to imagine removing a diseased native valve by catheter. Thus, these imaginative preliminary experiments are not yet directly relevant. We do not anticipate clinical application for many years. Catheter delivery of your artificial valve is *not* something you should take into consideration in any way at this time or for the foreseeable future.

How can you "repair" my valve? Wouldn't a brand new valve serve me better than a "rebuilt" one?

In certain cases, your own valve can be repaired rather than replaced. This is most applicable to the mitral valve. Repair is most relevant when the mitral valve is leaky rather than narrowed. In technical parlance, repair is often feasible for the condition of mitral regurgitation.

The development of the field of mitral valve repair represents one of the greatest advances in the history of cardiac surgery. This is largely the life's work of Dr. Alain Carpentier of Paris, France, one of the greatest surgeons in history, and arguably the best teacher of cardiac surgery *ever*.

Dr. Carpentier's techniques permit surgeons to excise the diseased portion of the mitral valve and bring the remaining tissues back together, with very delicate manipulation and suturing, to form a properly functioning whole. Usually the leak in the mitral valve results from tearing of one of the fine parachutelike chords that control the movement of the delicate mitral valve leaflets.

The segment of the mitral valve that is errant after the chord tears is removed, so that all remaining leaflet tissue is properly chord-supported. These events and procedures are illustrated in figure 12.8.

You are *not* being shortchanged if your mitral valve is repaired. There are major advantages to maintaining your own mitral valve. First, you shouldn't need Coumadin in the long term. This has its own advantages. Also, the fine chords that support your mitral valve also support the muscle of the left ventricle. There are advantages to the fact that this whole parachutelike apparatus is preserved when your mitral valve is repaired. Specifically, your heart muscle remains stronger because of this preservation, and your life expectancy is better in the long term.

On the other hand, some leaky valves just cannot and should not be repaired. In such a situation, a good valve replacement is better than an incomplete or nondurable valve repair.

For the aortic valve, repair techniques have not been generally adopted. Also, aortic valve replacement does not carry the detrimental consequences that can sometimes follow mitral valve replacement. For these reasons, repair is, practically speaking, limited to the mitral valve.

I don't feel that bad. Isn't it too early to replace my valve?

As the science of valve assessment and replacement becomes more and more advanced, we realize that in many cases, the left ventricle, the main pumping chamber of the heart, may be deteriorating even while the patient continues to feel well. This is especially true with the "leaky" conditions, mitral regurgitation and aortic regurgitation. If this deterioration progresses too far, the prospect of eventual surgery may become excessive, and the benefit may be limited, as the deterioration may be permanent, even after a new valve is placed. The reason is that the regurgitant lesions place a large-volume load on the left ventricle (see previous references to the Sisyphus-like burdens of leaky valves). The left ventricle stretches and stretches to keep an adequate amount of blood flowing forward despite the leaky valve. The stretched muscle is overloaded and suffers damage, both temporary and permanent.

Your doctor may recommend surgery, even if you feel well, if serial studies (usually ECHOs) show that your heart is progressively enlarging. This usually happens over time (months to years)

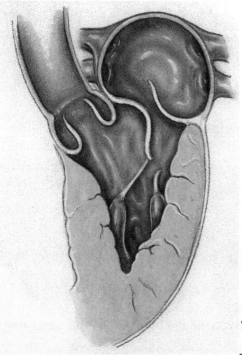

Figure 12.8. Chord of the mitral valve, courtesy of Edwards Lifesciences, Irvine, California. Note how the corresponding valve leaflet, no longer supported by the torn chord, has fallen back into the left atrium. This, of course, causes the valve to leak.

if the valve leakage is severe, causing the pumping of your chamber to stretch under the load. Likewise, if your studies show that the pumping strength of your left ventricle is falling, even to the lower ranges of normal, this is evidence of severe impact from your leaky valve. If your valve is not replaced promptly, your well-being and long-term survival will be compromised. Likewise, your doctor may do a stress test. If your left ventricle pumps more weakly under stress, that is an indicator that your heart is being

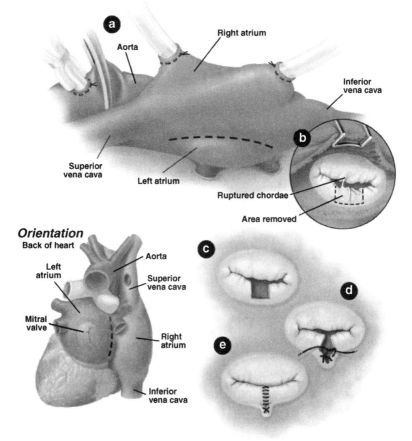

Figure 12.9. Mitral valve repair. Note the incision line in the left atrium that gives us access to the mitral valve. Note how we resect a rectangular portion of the leaflet that harbors the torn chord. Note how we reconstruct this delicate leaflet with sutures, to restore a properly functioning valve.

unduly damaged by the leaky valve. In such a circumstance, prompt surgery is vital.

In certain instances, your heart valve may be leaking so badly that surgery is recommended immediately, without serial studies. We grade the severity of leakage on a scale of I to II to III to IV. If you have grade IV leakage of your aortic or mitral valve, surgery will likely be recommended, as the outlook for this grade of severity is grim without surgical intervention.

Please also keep in mind that most patients with valvular heart disease learn to adjust to it. You may think you feel well, but you may have subtly limited your lifestyle and activities to adjust to your more limited heart capacity. You may take the elevator more than before, rather than walking the stairs. You may walk slowly rather than hustle. You may ride rather than walk around the golf course. Many patients tell us how very much better they feel with a new valve, even though they thought they felt "well" before.

Keep in mind also that your leaky heart valve is a *mechanical* problem. There is no medication that can make your valve function better. No amount of delay will make it function better. No medication can prevent the eventual damage of the leaky valve to your heart. A severely leaking heart valve is a *mechanical* problem that requires a *mechanical* solution. That solution is surgery.

Can't my valve be replaced by a robot?

Although robotic coronary artery bypass is in the early stages, robotic valve replacement is not currently feasible. Straightforward repairs of the mitral valve are, however, being attempted experimentally by robotic assistance. Perhaps in the next ten to twenty years, your valve replacement can be done through robotic means.

HEART TRANSPLANTS

I am just not eager to have a heart transplant. Aren't there any other operations you can perform to improve my heart function?

Many patients feel this way. It is probably safe to say that no patient looks forward to having his heart removed and having a new one put in its place. There are indeed dangers involved in this process. Also, there are some real changes in lifestyle after transplantation, including the need for immunosuppressive medications and routine surveillance biopsies.

On occasion, a conventional operation can forestall further cardiac damage and even restore some of the lost pumping strength. At Yale University, we have specialized in applying such techniques to patients with end-stage heart failure.

The operations that can be performed are four: coronary artery bypass surgery, aortic valve surgery, mitral valve surgery, and left ventricular aneurysmectomy. Each of these procedures is covered in detail in corresponding sections of this book. Here we will discuss their particular application to patients with advanced heart failure.

When a patient enters the hospital or begins an outpatient evaluation for advanced heart failure, we search diligently for any specific structural cause for this heart failure. Unfortunately, we often find no specific cause, and we end up attributing the weak pumping strength to an occult viral infection that occurred earlier in the patient's life. In some patients, however, we do find structural heart disease that has caused the weakening of the heart muscle.

If we find coronary artery disease; that is, blockage of the arteries of the heart, it is likely that the weak pumping strength of

Now, to follow up on the patients with valve disease from our prior vignettes:

Clark, the surgeon-colleague with mitral regurgitation, whom we met in chapter 4, underwent repair of his mitral valve about seven years ago. He has resumed his daily three-mile runs. Three of his four children are in college. The fourth is a senior in high school. Clark is completely well—asymptomatic, as we say in medical parlance. He takes no medications, not even Coumadin or aspirin.

Professor Voytek (chapter 3), the seemingly arrogant physicist, underwent replacement of his aortic valve with a biologic prosthesis, a pig valve. In the ensuing five years, he has continued to run three laboratories in different states. His work is progressing splendidly, although only a handful of the brightest of the bright can understand it. A Nobel Prize may be in the offering.

Angela, the attractive brunette (chapter 10), whose history of rheumatic fever so worried your author when he was a young man, continues very well. She has three children and has opened a maternity shop. She still has a murmur, but it does not trouble her in the least.

the heart is due to heart attacks. Although we cannot bring back heart muscle that has completely died in the heart attack, we can prevent future attacks by applying the coronary bypass operation. This should keep the strength of the heart relatively safe from future additional onslaughts. Also, there are nearly always some border zones on the edge of the completed heart attack areas where the heart muscle is impaired, but not dead, due to inadequate blood flow. Our clinical investigations, as well as those of others, have shown that we can *reanimate* these border zones via the coronary artery bypass operation.[3] It is not unusual for us to see even a ten-point improvement in the ejection fraction following the coronary bypass operation. Remember, a normal ejection fraction is about 60 to 70 percent.

Likewise, if the cause of the cardiac enlargement is a blocked or leaky aortic valve, surgery to replace that valve will take a tremendous load off the heart and almost always lead to considerable improvement in the pumping strength of the heart. With aortic valve disease, the improvements can be dramatic, and the outlook can be restored to a very good one.

If the cause of the weak pumping strength of the heart is a leaky mitral valve, corrective mitral valve surgery may also be of benefit. The likelihood of restoration of a good result is smaller here, but very worth pursuing in most cases.

If the cause of cardiac enlargement and weak pumping action is a left ventricular aneurysm, surgery to remove the aneurysm and remodel the heart to more normal contour and size can produce dramatic results. Pumping strength can be improved markedly. Long-term outlook, while not ideal, can be restored to a hopeful one. A state congresswoman who was in desperate straits before the operation and underwent aneurysm excision at our institution many years ago was able to return fully functional to her demanding schedule and remains well to this day.

Thus, if you have advanced heart failure, it is imperative to look for structural lesions as its cause. These may involve the arteries of your heart, or the valves, or an aneurysm of the left ventricle. Looking for such abnormalities will almost always involve an EKG, a cardiac ECHO, and, usually, a cardiac catheterization. These testing procedures are discussed fully in the pertinent sections of this book. If such structural lesions are found, a conventional operation may suffice as an alternative to transplantation. In fact, our research at Yale University has indicated that the outlook for patients treated with these more conventional operations, when applicable, equals or exceeds that with transplantation.

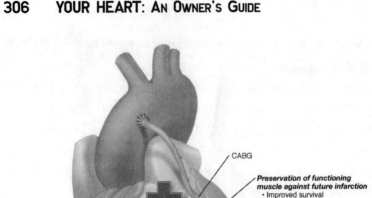

Figure 12.10. Reanimation of a heart attack zone by coronary artery bypass grafting. The lightning bolt signifies the reanimation of jeopardized heart muscle by the newfound blood flow after coronary bypass surgery. The red cross signifies the long-term protection of the remaining live muscle by virtue of the blood flow through the bypass grafts. EF stands for ejection fraction. CHF stands for congestive heart failure.

If no approachable structural lesions are found, however, transplantation may be the only surgical option.

Also, if you have already undergone a conventional operation in the past, especially the bypass operation, and you are being considered for cardiac transplantation, it is likely that no further conventional surgery will suffice.

How about those new operations I've heard about— the "splint" and the "sac" for the heart? Would those be of help for me?

Two new mechanical treatments for heart failure are being evaluated. One, the myosplint, actually skewers the left ventricle with rigid struts, aiming to restore a more natural and more powerful shape to the saggy, enlarged balloon of a heart that many patients with advanced heart failure develop.

Another mechanical treatment surrounds the heart with a lattice-like sac, called an Acorn cardiac support device, with the aim of preventing further dilatation of the heart. Dilatation is part of advanced heart failure and is very detrimental to the strength of cardiac contraction. Preventing or limiting dilatation could be beneficial.

Both of these treatments are entirely experimental. Initial clinical results are just coming in. While we need to have an open mind, it appears doubtful that either mode of therapy will become a breakthrough treatment.

How about the muscle wrap of the heart?

You have probably heard that cardiac surgeons are wrapping the heart with a large muscle borrowed from the back—the latissimus dorsi muscle—the muscle that gives weightlifters the triangular shape to the back. This is one of the strongest muscles in the human body. It was hoped that, by pacing this muscle to transform its biochemical characteristics to resemble heart muscle, heart function could be strengthened. Despite early enthusiasm, clinical results did not bear out major patient benefit. There is still hope for fashioning entire new accessory cardiac chambers from this muscle. This is much more complex an undertaking than simply wrapping the heart, but current research is limited in this field.

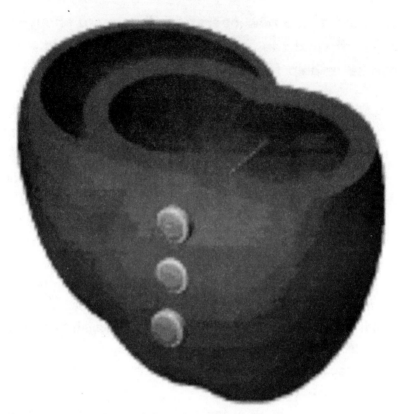

Figure 12.11. The myosplint device, courtesy of Myocor.

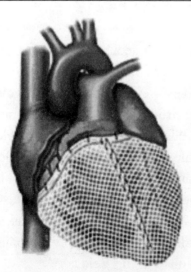

Figure 12.12. The acorn device,
courtesy of Acorn Cardiovascular

How about the Brazilian heart reduction operation?

Several years ago, a media frenzy was occasioned by a new operation for the dilated, weakened heart, originating from Dr. Rondas Battista of Brazil. This operation involves cutting out part of the wall of the left ventricle to bring down the diameter. Some of the glamour of this procedure stemmed from the paradox of cutting out live muscle from an already weakened heart. Despite initial enthusiasm, clinical research in the United States, Europe, and Japan found high risk and only modest benefit from this procedure. It has been virtually abandoned.

Am I too old for a transplant?

We used to say that sixty years was the strict upper-age limit for heart transplantation. This limit was in effect for two reasons: First, elderly patients did not do as well in the short or long term after heart transplantation. They died more frequently and had more complications. Second, there was a strong sense among doctors of an ethical imperative to allocate preciously scarce donor hearts to younger patients, who had not had an opportunity to live a full life.

Currently, the situation has changed somewhat, so that patients over sixty can, on occasion, be considered for transplantation. Certain high-profile cases have resulted in a consensus that strict age criteria are discriminatory and not acceptable. Also, results of transplantation in older patients have improved. So, if your general health, other than your heart, is good and you are active and have the potential for a vigorous life of good quality, you may be considered for transplantation even if you are over sixty. We are listing for transplantation more patients between sixty and sixty-five years of age. Beyond sixty-five, only the very rare patient will be considered for transplantation.

At Yale, we did a transplant on a very special patient, a stage actor and opera singer, who had been an athlete in his youth and was still in exceptional overall physical shape. He has since gone on to appear in multiple stage productions and operas in major metropolitan arenas. He has contributed to the artistic appreciation of many thousands of audience members since his transplant. We are certainly glad that we did not deny this individual transplantation solely on the basis of his age. He was sixty-seven then and is an active seventy-seven now.

I know donor organs are very scarce; will I live to get a transplant?

Your question is very well taken. Few hearts become available for transplantation. About three thousand patients are entered yearly in the United States on the transplant waiting list. Only one thousand organs become available yearly, and only one thousand of the three thousand waiting patients are actually transplanted. There appears little likelihood that this shortfall in available organs will improve at any time in the near future. In fact, the shortfall worsens each year as nontransplanted patients accumulate.

It is imperative that families have an awareness of the critical organ shortage and an open mind toward donation when death takes a loved one.

About 15 percent of patients waiting for a transplant die each year because no organ has become available for them.

How about animal hearts? Will we soon be able to transplant animal hearts into humans?

Famed transplant surgeon Dr. Norman Shumway of Stanford University was asked this question some years ago. Transplanting animal hearts is called *xenotransplantation* from the Greek word *xenos* meaning "stranger." Dr. Shumway's reply has become legendary. Xenotransplantation, he said, "is five years away. And it always will be." Clearly, Dr. Shumway did not feel that this modality was likely to come to clinical fruition.

The potential problems with such a procedure are numerous. First of all, the antigenic differences (differences in the immune "tags" on the outside of cells) between species will pose rejection dangers far exceeding those of human-to-human transplantation. Engineering nonantigenic animals is currently being attempted but is far from satisfactory as yet. There is also the serious potential danger of exposing the human race to infections, especially viruses, both known and unknown, which are currently limited to other species. Many experts consider this a serious concern, especially in the current AIDS era. Finally, there are ethical issues about growing genetically modified animals specifically for the purpose of donating their hearts to humans.

The regulation of research and application of xenotransplantation require the input of not only scientists but also of the clergy, ethicists, legislators, and the general public.

Is transplantation a dangerous operation?

Transplantation is actually much safer than you might have expected, especially for patients well enough to await the operation at home.

The current risk of death from transplantation is 10 percent. Conversely stated, 90 percent of patients will survive the transplant operation and the early recovery phase. About 80 percent to 90 percent of patients will be alive one year after transplantation.[4]

About 50 percent to 60 percent of transplantation patients will be alive five years later. After that point, it is quite likely that coronary artery disease will develop in the transplanted heart, leading to death over the five- to ten-year interval following transplantation. Some patients have lived over twenty years following transplantation, but that is the exception rather than the rule. These uniquely fortunate patients probably benefited from a fortuitously favorable immunologic match with the donor.

Fortunately, with modern antirejection medications, early death from rejection is rare. Every patient has rejection at some point, but this is usually very easily treated, and the patient is often not even clinically aware of this phenomenon. It is detected only by the routine surveillance biopsies of the heart.

Infection is a serious potential problem because the body's ability to combat infection is impaired by the antirejection medications. By use of preventive antibiotics, early removal of lines that can allow infection into the body, and careful surveillance, infection is less common than it was in the past.

One problem that medical science has not yet mastered—the virtual Achilles heel of clinical heart transplantation—is failure of the right side of the new heart, due to high pressures in the lungs. This problem, posttransplant right-heart failure, accounts for the vast majority of the early deaths after heart transplantation. Once the first week has passed, this problem no longer occurs.

Will you really take my new heart from a dead person?

The answer to your question is both yes and no.

The donor heart cannot ordinarily be taken from an individual who is dead in the usual sense—that is, without a heartbeat, pulse, or blood pressure. The heart is very sensitive to interruption of its own blood flow. If the donor were literally dead, his heart would not be of use. It would have died itself or become severely weakened.

However, the person whose family generously donates the heart for you will be dead in another sense—specifically, brain-dead. That is, although he will have a heartbeat, a pulse, and a blood pressure, he will be unconscious, without volitional movements, and certain never to attain consciousness again. Strict criteria have been developed for determination of brain death—to ensure that this declaration is accurate, unequivocal, and permanent.

Most donors have suffered some type of direct brain injury. This is most commonly from automobile or motorcycle accidents. Alternatively, the brain injury may occur from a gunshot wound to the head. In some cases, the brain is injured by rupture of a brain aneurysm. In all these cases, brain death will be diagnosed only after a rigid series of observations have been unequivocally confirmed by independent observers.

The wonder of transplantation is that it wrests great benefit out of the jaws of tragedy—made possible by compassion and generosity from the donor and/or his family.

How is the transplant operation done?

First, you are placed on the heart-lung machine, which substitutes for the pumping action of your heart. Then, your heart is removed. The first sight of the empty chest cavity is an encounter that no doctor ever forgets.

At the same time, the new heart arrives, usually brought by jet from the donor hospital. The new heart is trimmed and prepared to suit.

The new heart is attached to your body by a series of four anastomoses, or hookups. These are shown in the figure 12.13. These attachments include the left atrium, the right atrium, the aorta, and the pulmonary artery.

The new heart is allowed at least a half hour of blood flow after attachment to your body before it is given any load. At that point, in a gradual fashion, the burden of pumping your blood is transferred from the heart-lung machine to your new heart. Your new heart always needs some support with stimulating medications until it recovers from the trauma of excision, storage, and transportation.

How far away can you go to get my new heart?

The heart can last only four hours from the time it is removed to the time it is fully reimplanted in its new recipient. About one hour is required for the implantation itself. That leaves about three hours, maximum, for travel. If one includes ground travel time to and from the donor and recipient airports, say about one-half hour for both ends, that leaves about two and one-half hours for air travel. At the five hundred miles per hour that jets travel, that allows a range of just more than one thousand miles. That is why donor regions rarely exceed a one thousand mile-radius.

The entire entourage—surgeons, nurses, anesthesiologists, pilots, jet aircraft—are put into place solely to transport your new heart as quickly as possible. The jet is carrying your heart and your crew, and nothing else.

Why would my new heart be susceptible to heart failure? Didn't you pick my new heart to be strong?

This question is very well taken. You would not expect a new heart selected for its pumping strength to be vulnerable in any way. The truth is that the right side of the new heart is indeed vulnerable, at least for the first few days.

Remember that the right side of the heart pumps blood to the lungs; the left side pumps blood to the whole body. The right heart is much weaker and thinner-walled than the left.

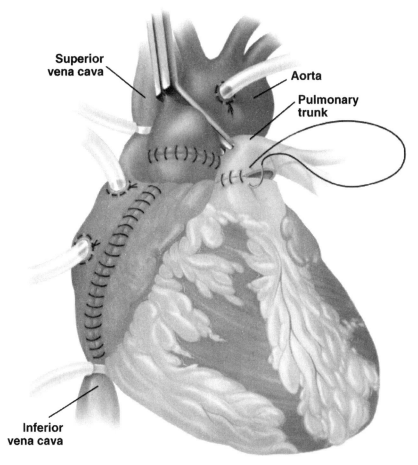

Figure 12.13. Heart transplantation. The last of four large suture lines is being completed. (One suture line lies behind the donor heart, out of view.)

Now, in the donor, the right heart pumps into healthy lungs—which are soft and not waterlogged. But once the new heart is transplanted into your body, it suddenly faces the great load of pumping into your lungs, stiff and waterlogged from months or years of congestive heart failure. The thin-walled right heart can fail, leading to low blood pressure or even death. Most early deaths after transplantation occur on this basis.

We use medications to support your new right heart for several days after transplantation. The muscle of the right heart adjusts quickly to its new burden.

This paradox of the struggling right heart is the reason that at Yale University we are developing a new heart transplant operation that preserves both your old right heart and your whole new heart, giving you double the strength on the right side. This procedure is still in development at the time of this writing.

Will transplantation transform my life?

The answer to this question is a resounding yes.

Predominantly, the changes will be for the better. You will have a new "motor," so your exercise capacity will greatly increase. After you recover from the surgery, you will probably feel better than you have for years. You will be able to breathe. You will no longer have that feeling that you are drowning from the fluid in your lungs. You will be able to walk as far as you like, without difficulty. You can even engage in sports, if you like. It will be as if your worn-out car's four-cylinder engine has been replaced with a Ferrari V-12 engine.

On the other hand, there are negatives. You will always be dependent on medications to prevent rejection. These are powerful drugs, and you will likely be on triple-drug therapy. Taking immunosuppressant medications means, in turn, that you will always be susceptible to infection. You will need to visit the hospital regularly, on an outpatient basis, for biopsies of your new heart, done via a short catheterization procedure. This is how we keep track of any rejection tendencies.

As time goes on, rejection and infection will become less likely. After you and your new heart have a year together, it is usually smooth sailing from that point on. And you have the reassurance that your life is not in jeopardy from moment to moment. Before your transplant, you probably had a very high chance of dying within six months. After your transplant, you are relatively secure. Your life expectancy is not normal, but the majority of patients will survive the next five years, a great boon by comparison to the chances without the transplant.

Will you be able to grow a new heart for me in the future?

Remarkably, tissue engineering techniques have succeeded in growing thin sheets of muscle cells that are actually *capable of contracting*. This is truly astounding. But it may take decades before these microscopic sheets can be collected into chunks of muscle that can contribute significantly to the mechanical function of the heart. Other problems have to do with developing a blood vessel network to nourish this new muscle and a nerve network to stimulate its contraction.

THE ARTIFICIAL HEART

Can you tell me something about the history of artificial heart use in human beings?

Artificial hearts have been used in humans since the 1960s. The Jarvik heart was tried in the early 1980s. The Jarvik heart replaced both the right and left sides of the heart. But a very important point is that in the vast majority of patients it is probably not necessary to replace both sides of the heart. As we discussed, most disease processes affect predominantly the left side of the heart, which needs to be very powerful. On the other hand, the right side of the heart pumps only to the lungs and does not need to be nearly as strong.

Patients given the original Jarvik heart model did not do well, mainly because of blood clots that formed in the device, leading to strokes. Since then, research has focused predominantly on replacing the left side of the heart alone. Two companies have developed left-side-only artificial heart devices. They are the Novacor and the HeartMate. Both are FDA-approved after nearly eighteen years of clinical experience. They are like Ford and Chevy, in that each has its supporters. The HeartMate is a little less prone to clots and strokes, while the Novacor (now called the WorldHeart) is a little more reliable.

Both the Novacor and HeartMate have a power cord that comes out through the skin and attaches to a small power pack roughly the size of a portable CD player. Patients with these devices can be very active, and the Novacor especially can last a long, long time. One of the patients at our institution has used the Novacor longer than any other American on any artificial heart device—three and a half years.

Wouldn't a nuclear power source be the obvious choice to supply the artificial heart? Wouldn't that eliminate the need for an external power cord?

This is a very good question. In fact, although the 80 watts or so that the artificial heart consumes is too much for an implanted battery, it would be "peanuts" for a small nuclear power source. Early research in the 1960s was headed in this direction.

It is little discussed, but the government quashed efforts aimed at achieving a totally implantable nuclear artificial heart. One con-

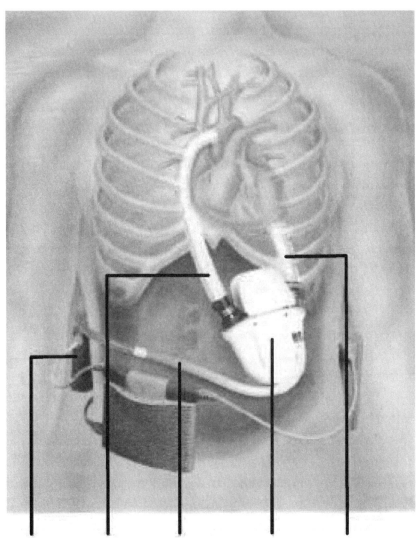

CONTROLLER AND POWER PACKS	OUTFLOW CONDUCT AND VALVE	PERCUTANEOUS LEAD	PUMP/DRIVE UNIT	INFLOW CONDUCT AND VALVE
Wearable external componants enable recipient mobility.	Carries blood from pump to ascending aorta.	Provides electrical connection and pump venting.	Implanted within anteior abdominal wall.	Carnulates left ventricular apex carries blood to pump.

Figure 12.14. The Novacor artificial heart device, courtesy of WorldHeart.

cern was that a terrorist might build a bomb by kidnapping and sac-
rificing dozens or hundreds of artificial heart patients for the purpose
of explanting their small uranium sources. No research on nuclear
power sources in medicine is being done at the present time.

Who needs an artificial heart?

At the present time, patients who are thought unlikely to survive the
many months on the waiting list usually necessary to secure a donor
heart are considered for an artificial heart.

As explained above, there are two artificial hearts in general
use at this time. Both replace the left side of the heart only, but that
suffices for the vast majority of patients in need. These two devices
are called the Novacor and the HeartMate. They are both capable
mechanical hearts—each with its own advocates and devotees.
These devices require a major operation for placement. Each has a
power cord that exits your skin. Both can be relied on to effectively replace your heart function for a long time. As noted, at
Yale, we have the longest-living American recipient of such a
device, who leads a very active life after three and a half years
with a Novacor device.

At a few centers, like ours, experimental trials are under way
using the Novacor and HeartMate not as bridges to transplantation,
as described above, but rather as destination, or permanent, therapies. The results are still being accumulated and analyzed.

A number of newer devices, smaller or without a power cord
exiting the body wall, are currently under testing. These include the
DeBakey/NASA device and the Jarvik 2000. These models may
come into use in the next several years if early beneficial data is
confirmed more widely.

A full, active life can be had with these artificial heart devices.
Patients can work, go to college, and engage in sports. The devices

can be noisy, however. Our longest-implanted patient, asked if he was bothered by the noise, answered, with a smile: "After all, what is the alternative?"

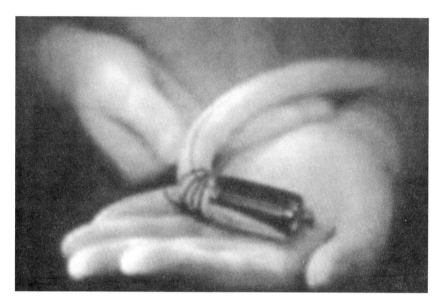

Figure 12.15. The Jarvik 2000 artificial heart device.

What about the AbioCor Heart?

The AbioCor, which has had a lot of press recently, represents another foray into complete, right and left heart replacement. There are two points to emphasize about the AbioCor: The first is that replacing both sides of the heart is unnecessary for most patients. To do so makes matters doubly complex when mechanical replacement of just the left side would suffice.

The second point is that the AbioCor does represent a major advance in one specific way: it does not have a power cord. Rather, energy is transmitted by radio frequency from a battery pack worn around the waist. Radio frequency technology for energy transmission for medical purposes originated at our own institution some thirty years ago. It was used by pioneer William W. L. Glenn for diaphragm pacing. AbioCor took the same technology and, quite appropriately, applied it to the artificial heart. This mode of energy transmission represents a major advantage, because the skin barrier does not need to be pierced by a power cord, thus dramatically lessening the risk of long-term infection.

Can a recipient actually feel the artificial heart inside him?

Yes, the devices are for the most part very large—bigger than your fist—and generate quite an impact when they fire. Both the bulk of the device, usually placed in the belly, and the jolt of contraction are very obvious—as is the mechanical noise. One of our patients was asked by a fellow patron in a movie theater, "Can't you turn that noisy thing off?" His answer was a simple "No."

What kinds of lifestyle changes do artificial heart recipients need to make?

Recipients can lead very active, nearly normal lives. They can go home from the hospital just one or two weeks after the implantation. But they do have to contend with the battery pack, which is always with them. The pack weighs several pounds. And blood thinners are usually required, as for an artificial heart valve. But the symptoms and limitations of heart failure that the recipient suffered before the artificial heart device was placed literally vanish. Instantly gone is the fluid accumulation, the shortness of breath, and the lack of energy with which the patient was previously plagued. It is as if the wheezing four-cylinder engine of a heart has suddenly been replaced with a Ferrari V-12.

Most of these devices cost about $80,000, and the hospitalization for their placement has a similar and additional cost.

What's on the horizon in artificial heart development?

The new generation of devices, unproven and just entering incipient clinical trials, are smaller. Some of the devices fit into the left ventricle itself. Mostly, they are driven by axial, screw-type impellers turning thousands of revolutions per minute, like turbines. It remains to be seen if they are safe and effective. These devices return once again to replacing the left side of the heart only. Soon, they should be available without power cords. Because of the shortage of hearts available for transplantation for end-stage heart failure, it is likely that artificial heart use will burgeon.

Now, to follow up on the patients from our clinical vignettes with heart failure:

David, the young track star profiled in chapter 2, got his new heart from a thirty-five-year-old woman. David is starting to run again. He is up to a mile. His best time so far after his transplant is six minutes. If it is up to him—and he is one determined young man— he will get his time down under five minutes, a record for a heart transplant patient.

Mr. Fulton (chapter 9), the insurance agent who decided to get the artificial heart, did indeed have this device placed. It served him very well—allowing him a full return to work, coaching, traveling, and the like. He lived with the device for three and a half years—a record for the United States. At that point, a heart became available for him. This courageous man lives a normal life today. With the support of his loving wife, he intends to swim the hundred-meter freestyle in the transplant Olympics. He is training daily.

Mr. Voytek, the arrogant self-proclaimed "VIP" whom we met in chapter 3, still waits for a donor heart. He has been in and out of the hospital for the last two years while awaiting a transplant. He is still intolerant of the fact that a heart cannot just be "made available" for him. His millions cannot make an organ appear or make it immunologically compatible with his system. Those issues are out of our human hands.

THE PERICARDIUM

Case 1. A Colleague in Trouble.

A colleague, a cardiologist, sat in front of your author's desk. He seemed perfectly well. But over a period of months, he had begun to develop swelling of his feet—edema, as it is called. And his belt line kept getting bigger and bigger, not from fat but from fluid in the abdomen. Also, his energy level was very low, and he became easily fatigued and occasionally light-headed.

A chest X-ray had shown calcium, or bony tissue, in the pericardium, the sac that encloses the heart. Calcium is very abnormal in that location, virtually sealing the diagnosis of *pericarditis*, or inflammation of the pericardial sac.

What is more, catheterization showed that pressures in all the heart chambers were very high, indicating that the irritated heart sac was shrinking down and literally squeezing the heart to death. That was why fluid was accumulating everywhere in his body, because it was backing up instead of being propelled through the heart. And his weakness, tiredness, and light-headedness were all due to the inability of the squeezed heart to generate sufficient forward flow of blood.

Why this had happened was not clear. Was it due to a virus? To undetected tuberculosis? To some radiation treatments the doctor/patient had had as a youngster?

It didn't much matter. Your author had to operate on his colleague, to strip the inflamed sac from the wall of the doctor's heart and remove it, thus releasing the stranglehold the heart sac had placed on that vital organ, the heart itself.

What is the pericardium?

The pericardium is a thin, glistening, flexible sac that surrounds the heart in the central chest. The pericardial space is normally lubricated by a small amount of fluid, called *pericardial fluid*.

Although it is thin and flexible (bendable), the pericardium is very inelastic (unstretchable). If excess fluid accumulates in the pericardial space, the pericardium does not stretch. Because the pericardium does not stretch, the excess fluid can put pressure on the heart, with serious consequences.

What is pericarditis?

Pericarditis is an inflammation of the pericardium. Remember that *inflammation* is the technical term for irritation. So, in pericarditis, the pericardium becomes irritated.

You have probably had an irritated eye at some point, with redness, tearing, and engorgement of the blood vessels in the white of the eye. Inflammation of the pericardium is very similar; the normally white-colored pericardium becomes irritated, swollen, and reddened, with engorged blood vessels in its wall.

The inflammation of the pericardium can, on occasion, represent a true infection. Rarely, this may be due to bacteria. More commonly, this is due to viruses, and can accompany a cold or a flu syndrome.

What happens if a person develops pericarditis?

Most cases of pericarditis are very mild. Your doctor may hear a rubbing noise when he listens to your heart, representing friction between the irritated membranes as the heart twists within the pericardial sac. Usually, antibiotics are not prescribed, as only rarely is a bacterium the cause. (Antibiotics do not fight viruses, they combat only bacteria.) Your doctor may prescribe anti-inflammatory medications to decrease the irritation of the membranes and encourage resolution of the state of irritation.

At times, the pericarditis may cause undo buildup of fluid in the pericardial space. The fluid may need to be drained by a needle. This procedure is called *pericardiocentesis*. If this is done, the opportunity exists to send the fluid for analysis to determine its cause. Usually, no specific cause is identified, and we conclude, by exclusion, that the irritation was due to a virus. Occasionally, pericarditis is due to tuberculosis—yes, the same germ that can affect the lungs. This is, of course, much less common than it was decades ago. At times, the pericarditis may be due to an immune reaction within the body, with no infection at all.

If the fluid accumulation is severe, or if the fluid returns after being removed by needle, surgery is performed. This surgery involves not only removing the fluid directly but also removing the pericardium itself, so that the syndrome can never recur. This procedure is called *pericardiectomy*. Removal of the pericardium provides ample material for microscopic analysis of the tissue in the pathology laboratory. This analysis may reveal the cause of the problem.

Wait just a minute. How can you remove my pericardium? Didn't Nature put it there for a reason?

This question is very well taken. Most or all of the structures in the human body perform very important functions. In the case of the pericardium, however, its removal has absolutely no adverse consequences. In fact, in case of large pericardial effusion (fluid collection around the heart, within the heart sac), failing to remove the pericardium could result in fatality. You will feel no difference whatsoever compared to when you still had a pericardium; you will not even know it is gone.

What is pericardial tamponade?

If the amount of fluid in the heart sac increases too much or too quickly, the heart becomes compressed—due to the inelasticity, or inability to stretch, of the pericardial sac. When the heart is squeezed by external fluid, the heart chambers are prevented from filling. Because the chambers cannot fill properly, the heart cannot pump blood effectively. A state of low-forward flow from the heart results—known technically as *low cardiac output syndrome*. This can make you weak or dizzy, or actually lead to shock or death if undetected and unattended.

This condition of excess fluid around the heart, which impairs the pumping function of the heart, is known as pericardial tamponade.

Pericardial tamponade can be caused by a large pericardial effusion. The appropriate treatment is pericardiectomy. Pericardiectomy means surgical removal of the pericardium.

Pericardial tamponade can also occur after cardiac surgery. If this happens, it usually occurs during the first night after the operation. If bleeding develops from a surgical site—the connections of the bypass grafts or the sites where the tubes of the heart-lung machine were connected, for example—the bloody fluid may accumulate in the pericardial space. Usually, this fluid will be evacuated through the drains left alongside the heart; occasionally, though, the accumulation may be too great to be accommodated by the drainage tubes. In such a case, serious impairment of heart function may occur. Even shock may ensue.

Pericardial tamponade from bleeding is one of the main conditions for which you will be monitored after cardiac surgery by your nurses and doctors. It will usually be detected well in advance of the time when any detriment to your heart function would become manifest.

If you do develop pericardial tamponade from postoperative bleeding, you will need to be "re-explored." As the term implies, a second-look procedure is performed to evacuate the clots from around your heart and determine if any surgical site is still bleeding. If so, an additional stitch or two may be placed. This can happen even at the most expert medical centers. In fact, up to one in twenty patients may require re-exploration. Believe it or not, usually no active bleeding site is identified. Re-exploration is usually quick, effective, and well tolerated—although intrinsically frightening to the family and loved ones of the patient.

If you think about it, it is amazing that postoperative bleeding does not occur in every patient. We place stitches very carefully in the vessels being attached—often dozens of individual sutures. Yet, in between the stitches are spaces, spaces through which blood can, in principle, leak. Wondrous Nature seals these spaces with microscopic deposits of clot material and a healing tissue called fibrin. Every now and then, the combination of surgical precision and Nature's helping hand does not suffice, and bleeding results.

How about *pericardial constriction*? What is that?

Rarely, months or even years after an episode of pericarditis, the heart sac can become thickened and inflexible, at times even contracted. Just try to imagine the consequences of having the heart sac squeeze down on your heart. The heart sac, in these cases, virtually chokes the heart. Severe heart failure results. Surgery is required. This is a serious operation, as the heart sac sometimes fuses with the outer layer of the heart, resulting in a difficult and dangerous plane for surgical dissection. Nonetheless, at experienced institutions like ours, surgery for pericardial constriction is generally safe and extremely effective. Normal heart function is restored.

Now, for some follow-up on the cardiologist in the vignette at the beginning of this section. We removed his pericardium, which was exceedingly difficult. Unexpectedly, we found he also had suffered heart attacks over the years, and needed bypasses as well. His heart was very weak going into the operation, and he was very, very sick in the first hours after return to ICU. In fact, at one point, his heart stopped, and your author needed to do CPR. The heart started back up, he recovered progressively and fully, and in the last eight years has gone on to even greater professional accomplishments and distinctions.

ANEURYSMS

Isn't surgery to remove an aneurysm too risky?

Although this is a big operation, it is generally safe in the present day, when done in what we call an *elective*, or nonurgent, planned fashion. At centers like ours, most aneurysms in the ascending aorta can be removed with a mortality risk of about 2 to 3 percent. For aneurysms of the descending aorta, the risk of mortality is closer to 8 percent. For aneurysms of the abdominal aorta alone, for which the heart-lung machine is not required, the risks are even lower than for the ascending aorta.

There is also a risk of stroke from these operations, usually due to liberation of debris from the aneurysm into the brain. This can occur despite the tremendous precautions that we take during the operation. The likelihood of stroke is about 8 percent. Of course, the exact expectation varies greatly, depending on your age, the location of your aneurysm, and the degree of arteriosclerosis and debris in your aorta.

For operations on the descending aorta, but not others, paraplegia can occur. This represents paralysis of the legs, which can be permanent. This occurs in about 10 percent of such operations, as critical blood vessels supplying the spinal cord may have arisen from the replaced segment of aorta. This problem has proved insoluble, despite a concerted effort by researchers in this area.

These risks may sound formidable, and indeed they can be, but they must be weighed against the likelihood of death from the aneurysm itself, which, for symptomatic, large, or growing aneurysms, can be extremely great. Without an operation, the natural risk of devastating aneurysm-related events is 15 percent for even moderately large aneurysms (six centimeters in diameter or more). The other factor to keep in mind is that operation for aortic aneurysm is much, much safer when done as a planned procedure under controlled circumstances, rather than in an emergency when the aneurysm is leaking or ruptured.

Your doctor will advise you on the relative risks and benefits of surgery for your particular aneurysm. We find that patients fall into two patterns. Some prefer to avoid potentially risky surgery, taking a "we'll see what time brings" approach regarding potential rupture. Other patients, the majority, feel they need to have the "time bomb" represented by the aneurysm extirpated as soon as possible, as they cannot emotionally tolerate living in such a vulnerable state.

PACEMAKERS

Who needs a pacemaker?

For some patients, their heart rate may be too slow at baseline or may fall too low at specific isolated times. In general, we like to see a heart rate between sixty and one hundred beats per minute at rest.

Remember that the forward output of the heart is dependent on the heart rate. Generally, the faster the heart rate, the larger the forward output of the heart. By corollary, if the heart rate falls too low, the output of the heart will be insufficient.

Very few of us, with the exception of trained athletes, can maintain a good forward cardiac output at heart rates below sixty beats per minute. Thus, this represents the lower range of heart rates at which we become concerned. In fact, there is a special term for heart rates below sixty: *bradycardia*, which means "low heart rate."

If your heart rate falls below sixty, it is quite possible that you may need a pacemaker. This is especially true if you have symptoms related to this low heart rate, such as dizziness, passing out, or severe lack of energy. If you have these symptoms and demonstrate sustained or episodic bradycardia, you likely need a pacemaker. The pacemaker can be absolutely lifesaving for you. A very low heart rate can easily and frequently be fatal. So dramatic can be the loss of consciousness related to a sudden slow heart rate that the medical term *drop attack* has been coined. That is to say, with a sudden onset of low heart rate, the patient loses consciousness and literally drops to the ground like a sack of potatoes.

You may hear your doctor talk about various types of slow heart rates. First is *sinus bradycardia*; this means a low heart rate that originates in the sinus node, the heart's internal pacemaker.

Alternatively, your doctor may tell you that you have *first-degree heart block*; this refers to a slight delay in conduction of electrical impulses in your heart.

More serious is *second-degree heart block*, in which some beats are actually dropped.

Most serious is *third-degree* or *complete heart block*, in which all normal beats are blocked. In such a rhythm, your heart stops unless an internal accessory pacemaking tissue in your heart jumps into action—which does not always occur.

How is a pacemaker placed?

Placement of a pacemaker is usually a quick, straightforward process. That is not to say it is trivial, but it usually goes extremely smoothly and involves little or no discomfort for you. You are sedated but not fully anesthetized. Novocain is injected just under your collarbone and a small incision is made. One of the veins that leads to your heart is accessed, and the pacing lead is passed through that vein and positioned carefully at the tip of your right ventricle, directly inside your heart. The position is checked carefully by X-ray, and the electrical characteristics of pacing are calculated to be sure that they are optimal. A small pocket is fashioned to accommodate the pacing unit, and the incision is closed.

Pacemakers generally last eight to twelve years or more. Living with a pacemaker should be imperceptible to others and have minimal or no adverse impact on your quality of life. In fact, in patients who need them, pacemakers are essential for preservation of life.

Chapter
13
AFTER SURGERY

POSTOPERATIVE RESTRICTIONS

Should I engage a private-duty nurse to care for me after surgery?

This is a frequently asked question. When you are in intensive care, no private-duty nurses are generally allowed. The nursing skills required are very advanced and specialized, and the nurses in that unit have been specifically selected and trained for those purposes. Also, while you are in intensive care, you will automatically receive one-to-one or one-to-two care. So, no private-duty nurses are needed or permitted while you are in intensive care.

When you graduate to the regular floor, the staff hospital nurses can tend to all your fundamental physiologic needs (pulse, blood pressure, urine output, fluid balance, and the like) and to the administration of your medications. With the decrements in staffing of recent years, however, they may not be able to attend to all of your creature comforts promptly and to subtleties of your recovery. A private-duty nurse can be very beneficial, if your means allow it, during the days that you are on the regular floor. The private-duty nurse can also help with meals, with getting you to and from the bathroom, and with the all-important process of getting you to walk.

Walking is the key to a good recovery. Walking keeps the blood flowing in your legs, which prevents formation of clots. Walking expands your lungs and cleanses the breathing passages. Walking helps your intestines to wake up, so that you resume your appetite and bowel movements, and it helps your bladder to awaken, so that you can void your urine on your own.

If your means do not permit private-duty nurses, who can be very expensive, just having family members around can help tremendously with meals, bathroom needs, and ambulation.

How will I feel when I wake up? What tubes will be in place at that time?

This photograph shows a patient just out of the operating room in the cardiac surgical ICU. This should not be frightening to you. All the apparatus shown in this picture is standard.

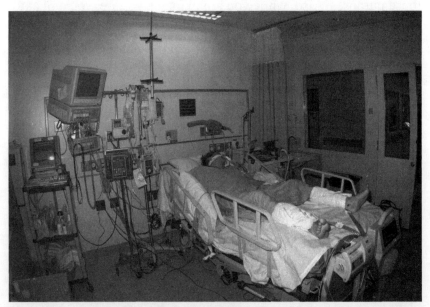

Figure 13.1. A recovering postoperative cardiac surgical patient. Do not worry— this patient did fine, despite all the intimidating equipment shown in the photo.

The breathing tube passes through the mouth into the trachea, or windpipe. This tube is necessary because early after surgery is completed, you are still not awake enough to breathe on your own. This tube is irritating and can elicit a strong gag, like when your throat is checked with a tongue depressor. However, the patient generally remains quite sedated while the tube is in place. The patient is allowed to awaken for about an hour while the tube is still in place, so that he can demonstrate that he is breathing adequately on his own. The large yellow IV in the right side of the neck is the Swan-Ganz catheter, which is used to measure pressures in the various heart chambers, to measure the pumping effectiveness of the heart, and to administer potent medications that may be necessary. The three large tubes exiting the bottom of the chest are the drains that remove excess fluid from around the heart and lungs for about forty-eight hours after surgery. The fine electrical wires near the bottom of the chest are the pacing wires, which all patients receive to permit control of heart rate early after surgery. The chest tubes are usually removed the morning of the second day after surgery, and the wires are removed the day before discharge. The special IV at the left wrist is the *arterial* line; this actually goes in a small artery, rather than a vein, so that your blood pressure can be monitored continuously from beat to beat. Also, arterial blood is harvested (painlessly) from that line so that your oxygen level can be measured. The yellow catheter near the groin is the Foley catheter, which drains urine from the bladder continuously. It is mildly uncomfortable to place this urinary catheter, but it is inserted after you are already asleep and in the operating room. It will be removed around the morning of the second day. Its removal is nearly painless. Monitoring the level of urine output hour by hour is one of the most important means of assessing your circulatory state.

What is displayed on the monitor beside my ICU bed, and why is the alarm going off repeatedly? Am I in trouble?

The alarm by your bedside—the heart monitor—tracks a number of your important cardiac and respiratory functions while you are in ICU (see figure 13.2).

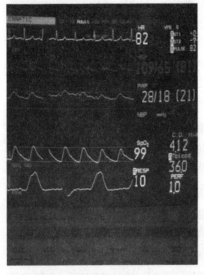

Figure 13.2. The bedside cardiac monitor. This displays blood pressure and other valuable parameters from instant to instant.

These functions include the following:

EKG. One tracing, usually the top one, displays your EKG, or electrocardiogram. This allows the nurse and doctors to know the rate and rhythm of your heart. We like to see a heart rate somewhere between 60 and 120 beats per minute. Rates outside this range usually are deleterious and need to be treated.

Blood pressure. Another trace shows your blood pressure, monitored continuously in real time from a special IV in a small artery in your wrist. This is a very important tracing. If you should go into shock, bleed, develop a fluid collection around the heart, or have a serious heart attack or arrhythmia, your blood pressure would fall. Having this tracing of your blood pressure permits immediate detection and correction of these potentially very serious conditions. We like to see your blood pressure between 80 and 140 millimeters of mercury (mmHg) systolic pressure.

Lung pressure. Another trace shows the pressure measured via your pulmonary artery catheter. This catheter sits in the inside of your heart, with its tip in the main pulmonary artery, the large blood vessel that leads directly into your lungs. The pressure in your lungs is much lower than the blood pressure, because the lungs are "softer" than the other organs in your body. This pressure usually runs 20 to 30 or 40 systolic. This catheter also displays exactly how many liters of blood your heart is pumping. The nurse makes an injection into the catheter, and a few seconds later the monitor gives the output reading for your heart. We like to see your heart pumping three to five liters of blood per minute for women, and four to six liters of blood per minute in men. (Remember, a liter is about one quart.)

Oxygen level. Another trace shows how full, or *saturated*, your blood is with oxygen. This is measured by a clip-on probe placed on the tip of one of your fingers. Normally, your blood is 95 percent or more saturated with oxygen. If the saturation falls below 90 percent, this can be serious and needs to be rectified.

Beside each of these tracings, usually to the right, you will see a numerical display of the parameter measured by that particular trace—be it heart rate, blood pressure, pulmonary artery pressure, or oxygen saturation.

Now, about those alarms that go off almost all the time: Most are completely spurious. Any of a number of common monitoring problems can cause the corresponding alarm to sound. If your EKG "sticky pads" come loose from your skin, the EKG alarm will sound. If you move, the EKG can detect the electrical activity of your muscles and erroneously interpret this as a rapid arrhythmia. In fact, the act of brushing one's teeth can look deceptively like ventricular tachycardia—we brush at the same rate as the heart races in this serious arrhythmia. The oxygen saturation monitor is especially temperamental. It will read falsely unless it is perfectly positioned. The nurse usually needs to adjust this frequently.

All the bells and whistles that sound under these false alarm scenarios are of no consequence. Your nurse can tell immediately that this is the case. In fact, the overwhelming majority of alarm triggerings are false.

Every now and then, the alarm indicates a bona fide aberration. Your nurse will be able to tell this immediately when she checks out the cause of the alarm. If the aberration is true, she will institute corrective action.

Again, remember—and emphasize this to your family—only one in hundreds or thousands of the alarm soundings of your bed-side monitor is likely to be a true one. You can relax, secure in the knowledge that your medical professionals are watching for the rare true alarm condition.

What is this breathing exercise machine the nurse placed on my bedside table?

Keeping your lungs clean and well expanded is a vital part of your recovery. The machine by your bedside is called an *incentive spirometer*. This machine, which comes in several commercial forms, is designed to force you to take a deep breath. With one commercially available device, the stronger you inhale, the more of the three weighted balls you are able to lift up. When you reach the stage where you can raise the third ball, then you can try to keep it afloat even longer.

You should work on this instrument five minutes per hour every waking hour. In so doing, you will combat the natural collapse (*atelectasis*) to which your lungs are prone after major surgery. You will also clear your airways of the phlegm that builds up after anesthesia and surgery. The result will be that you will avoid pneumonia and lung collapse.

Why did the nurse ask me to flap my feet every hour?

After major surgery, patients are prone to develop clots in the large veins of the legs. This is known as deep vein thrombosis. This is very dangerous because these clots can travel to the lungs, producing a blockage in the lungs known as a *pulmonary embolism*. This can be life-threatening or even fatal.

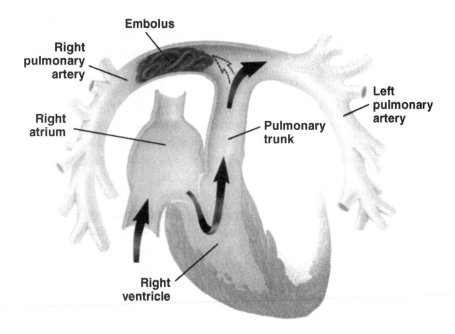

Figures 13.3. Illustration of an embolus of the pulmonary artery caused by deep vein thrombosis. A blood clot from a deep leg vein has reached the lung.

By flapping your foot up and down repetitively, you pump blood through the veins in your legs. This mimics the flow characteristics of an active lifestyle with frequent walking. By keeping the blood moving in your leg veins, you will forestall deep vein thrombosis and pulmonary embolism.

Can I shower?

There is some variation in surgeons' feelings about timing of the first shower, but all would agree that you can shower after you go home, if not before.

Should I put creams or salves on my wound?

We generally do not advocate that any cream or other substance be placed on your wounds, which will heal naturally without such supplements. Some surgeons recommend that a cream containing vitamin E be started a week or two after surgery, when the wound is completely sealed. This may improve the appearance of the scar that will form.

What kind of care will I need after discharge? Skilled nursing facility? Visiting nurse? Home health aide?

In the absence of specific problems with your wounds or pulse rate or breathing, you will probably not require any specialized care. Most patients can go directly home as long as a friend or family member is available most of the time for about a week to help with the activities of daily living. You may well need help getting around the house, showering, and certainly cooking, cleaning, and shopping. Many elderly patients find they need help especially at night, when they may manifest some residual confusion or need help navigating about the house in the dark. In most cases, you will be nearly independent by about one week after returning home, and your friend or family member will no longer need to be in attendance.

If there are wounds that need specialized care, the visiting nurse can usually come once or at most twice a day to assist in application of dressings. He may also take your pulse and blood pressure and listen to your heart and lungs, but this is not usually necessary for most patients. A home health aide may be arranged for several hours a day to help in the activities of daily life if no family member is available full-time. Individual insurance carriers may or may not cover this option.

These days, people lead busy lives and may not have a discretionary week to spend with the recovering heart surgery patient. In such a case, it is best to spend one to two weeks at an out-of-hospital extended nursing facility.

What will be my restrictions after surgery? When can I drive?

You will generally be asked to avoid heavy lifting to allow your wound(s) to heal. We usually advise not lifting anything heavier than a gallon of milk. This is to protect your sternotomy incision from compromise. However, mild aerobic activity is fine. We encourage you to walk every day—outdoors, if weather permits. You will easily become short of breath at first, but your exercise capacity will increase gradually over four to six weeks. By the time of your one-month postoperative visit to your surgeon, it would be ideal if you were walking one mile five or more days per week. This may not be feasible for all patients, especially those with arthritis or vascular disease of their legs. Complete wound healing takes about six months, but by the three-month point, there is plenty of strength, even in your breastbone, for you to do anything you wish. At that stage, you can lift anything your general condition and health allow.

We usually advise refraining from driving for one month. We encourage you, however, to ride in a car from the time you are discharged. Please do wear your seatbelt! There are two reasons to avoid driving yourself: We do not want you to stress your incision by turning the wheel or shifting the transmission. These concerns may be less urgent than they were in the past, before the near-universal advent of power steering and automatic transmissions. The second reason is to prevent you from injuring someone else on the road, in the event you get a sudden pain that affects your use of arms or legs.

Climbing stairs is fine. There is no need to move your bed to the first floor. The aerobic activity of climbing stairs is good for you. Just be careful not to fall. Also, be aware that the stairs will be quite an aerobic challenge for you at first.

We want you to be as active as possible within these mild restrictions. Go out shopping. The mall is a good place to walk in inclement weather. Go out to dinner. Go to a movie or a play. Do not be a recluse. Family members: Do not baby the recovering heart surgery patient.

What about sex?

Sexual activity is fine as soon as you return home and feel up to it. We prefer that you refrain from it while you are still in the hospital! (An occasional couple have failed to heed this restriction.) Sexual activity is quite safe and represents good aerobic exercise. Feel free to partake. You may find that certain positions are more comfortable than others until your wounds heal, but we would not impose any restrictions other than those dictated by comfort. The emotional benefits of the return to sexual relations can be considerable for both partners. Go ahead and enjoy.

What should I watch for after discharge? When should I call my doctor or return to the hospital?

In most cases, your common sense is the best guide. If you are not dizzy or light-headed, if you are breathing relatively comfortably, if you do not feel markedly feverish, and if you do not have unusual or copious drainage from your wounds, chances are very good that there is nothing significantly wrong that needs further attention. You do not need to take your pulse or temperature or blood pressure regularly unless so instructed by your medical team.

If you do feel feverish, you should take your temperature. A temperature no higher than 101 degrees Fahrenheit is considered normal.

If you are feeling light-headed, you or your family member can take your pulse at the wrist, in the groin, or at the neck. Rates greater than 60 beats per minute and less than 120 beats are normal. Rates below 60 or above 120 should be reported immediately.

If you have a blood pressure machine, you can take your pressure if you are feeling light-headed. If the systolic pressure, the top number, is above 90 mmHg and below 160 mmHg, that is normal. Pressures outside these limits should be reported immediately.

If you have passed out, have severe chest pain like that before surgery, or are dizzy, you should call an ambulance immediately and proceed to the emergency room of your hospital, or at least contact your care team. If you have lost consciousness for any reason, your family should call the ambulance. The same is true if you have a seizure or have onset of paralysis or severe numbness of a limb or have difficulty articulating words. These findings could signal a postoperative stroke. Sudden, curtainlike loss of vision in one eye is another important sign. All these symptoms warrant a call for an ambulance or at least a call to your care team.

If you develop significant redness or inflammation (irritation) at the sites of your incisions, this should be reported to the care team. Likewise, if you have drainage from your wounds, this should be reported. A small amount of thin bloody drainage from your leg wound is very common, but yellow, white, or puslike drainage from either your leg wound or your chest wound should be reported promptly. This drainage may signify an infection requiring treatment.

If you have a weight gain exceeding three pounds or if you develop swelling of both ankles or feet, this may be a sign of excess fluid retention or congestive heart failure. This should be reported to your team. Some swelling of the leg from which the vein was harvested is normally seen in all patients; usually the opposite leg, however, is not affected.

The vast majority of patients have no problems whatsoever after discharge. The problems mentioned above are uncommon. The bottom line is, if you are feeling fine, things are generally fine, and your care team will be happy.

What is this "fibrillation" that my friend had after his bypass?

There are two kinds of fibrillation of vastly different significance. Fibrillation represents a chaotic, constant, irregular heartbeat. You can return to chapter 3, figure 3.1, to view representative tracings of patients' electrocardiograms that illustrate a variety of heart rhythms, including a normal rhythm (in the jargon, *normal sinus rhythm*), atrial fibrillation, and ventricular fibrillation.

When the lower, powerful, pumping chambers of the heart fibrillate, that is called *ventricular fibrillation*. This is a very serious condition, causing loss of consciousness and cardiac arrest. Still, this is very uncommon after cardiac surgery. This requires defibrillation, the administration of a powerful electrical shock with the paddles, as is commonly portrayed on television medical shows.

When the upper, less important, pumping chambers of the heart fibrillate, that is called *atrial fibrillation*, which is relatively benign. About one in eight patients beyond the age of eighty have atrial fibrillation as their normal rhythm. After cardiac surgery, for reasons that even the experts do not understand, almost 40 percent of patients develop atrial fibrillation within the first several weeks. This is a nuisance, but not a serious concern. You may or may not sense a rapid, irregular heartbeat. Your heart rate may initially be as high as 150 or 160 beats per minute. The nurses and doctors will promptly come into your room with an EKG machine and possibly a temporary external pacemaker. It seems like a major event, but this is really quite routine. The team will start to adjust medications with the aim of bringing your heart rate down below 125 beats per minute; this level of control may take multiple adjustments over one or two days or more. You must not mistake these events for a serious turn in your condition. Atrial fibrillation after cardiac surgery is a benign development that you should expect during your recovery. If you don't have it, you are among those patients lucky enough to be spared this nuisance.

Should I resume my preoperative medications when I return home?

This is an important question, and the answer is a resounding no!

Your medications will have changed considerably after your operation. You may take some of the same or similar medications as before, but you should not start these on your own. You should take only what is prescribed for you at the time of hospital discharge. Some medications needed before for your angina may be eliminated by virtue of the operation itself. You may now be placed on anticoagulants, which you were not taking before. You will need medications to treat or prevent the rapid heart rhythm, called atrial fibrillation, which occurs after the operation. You may start taking water pills. Your blood pressure may require less, or more, treatment after surgery—at least in the short term.

You should take only and explicitly those medications prescribed for you by the surgical team at the time of your discharge from the hospital. You will receive a written list of new prescriptions. Often, your medical cardiologist will have made recommendations that have been incorporated into determining your discharge medications. You should completely disregard your preoperative medications. To mix and match between what you were taking before and what is newly prescribed would be very dangerous, quite possibly life-threatening.

POSTOPERATIVE MEDICATIONS

What medications will I take after discharge?

Years ago, surgeons hoped that the bypass operation would eliminate the need for cardiac medications. We no longer strive toward this goal, for newer evidence indicates that cardiac patients benefit from long-term administration of certain types of drugs.

There is evidence that the class of drugs known as beta-blockers leads to improved survival in cardiac patients. They decrease your heart rate, thus limiting the strain on your heart. You were probably taking these medications to control your angina before surgery. After the bypass operation, it is likely that your angina will be gone; however, your doctors will continue prescribing beta-blockers to provide long-term survival benefit.

Many patients with coronary artery disease take lipid-lowering drugs to control the levels of fatty substances in their blood. These will still be necessary after your operation. The bypass operation is plumbing—delicate and precise, but plumbing nonetheless. It does not change the chemistry of your body. The control of your cholesterol and triglycerides will continue to be vital, so that you can gain maximum benefit over time from your bypass.

Many cardiac patients suffer from preexisting hypertension, or high blood pressure. The cardiac operation does not permanently change your blood pressure. Although the pressure may be a bit higher or a bit lower during your hospitalization, it will return to your preoperative pattern. You will need to continue your blood pressure medications.

Many cardiac surgical patients have diabetes. You will need to continue your diabetic medications after surgery, be they oral agents or insulin. Please be aware that your medication requirements will vary around the time of your operation. Remember that hypoglycemia—abnormally low blood sugar—is a bigger potential problem for surgery patients than hyperglycemia—abnormally high blood sugar level. We will aim to keep your blood glucose (sugar) levels in the high 100s or low 200s. After you are home and your appetite has returned, you and your doctor will resume the stricter control that you exercised before.

Many patients are on Coumadin, a blood thinner used for atrial fibrillation, before the operation. This heart rhythm is very common, especially after age seventy-five. You will still need your Coumadin after surgery. Even patients who did not have atrial fibrillation before the operation may develop this rhythm after surgery—a full 40 percent, in fact, even in young patients. You will go home on a variety of medications to control this rhythm, usually including Coumadin.

In addition, you may need to start Coumadin if you have had valve surgery, as many artificial valves require blood thinners to prevent blood clots and related problems. (These issues are covered in chapter 12 in the section titled "Valve Replacement.")

REHABILITATION

What about a cardiac rehab program?

Many medical centers have excellent cardiac rehabilitation programs. Your cardiologist will advise you on his recommendations. Formal cardiac rehab probably will not start until one to two months after surgery. If you are a coronary artery bypass patient, your cardiologist may have you do an exercise test, also known as a treadmill test or stress test, before clearing you to engage in formal rehab. These programs are usually very helpful, not only physically but also emotionally. Many patients become attached to the rehab staff with whom they work regularly.

If you do not have access to a rehab program, you can certainly do the rehabilitation on your own. Walking is the key. You can start right after the operation. Walking will be difficult at first; you will get short of breath with minimal effort, but your stamina will improve progressively. If you are married, you and your spouse can walk together; this is an opportunity for postoperative bonding. Walking with a friend is an excellent way to stay in touch. If you are walking at least one mile five days a week, your surgeon will be very pleased by the time of your one-month visit. (Be advised that this goal may not be attainable for those with noncardiac restrictions, such as hip disease, so common in the elderly.) The local mall is a great place to walk in case of inclement weather. Your authors, in fact, often find that visiting the mall is like holding office hours—our patients abound. Not uncommonly, patients find us and present their questions as well as display their surgical wounds. Treadmills and exercise bicycles are excellent alternatives to walking.

SPECIFIC CONDITIONS

A friend told me he could "hear" his heartbeat after his bypass operation. Will this bother me?

Many patients have told us that they are very aware of their heartbeat after the operation. They can often hear the heartbeat at night in a quiet room, especially as they lay their head on a pillow. They may also sense that their heartbeat is stronger, more powerful, after the operation.

First, this sensation is not at all dangerous. Second, the increased awareness of the heartbeat will very likely lapse slowly over time.

We do not know why patients have this increased awareness of their heartbeat. In some cases, the beat is actually stronger, as perceived. In certain cases, the blocking medications, which decrease the strength of the heartbeat, have been decreased or eliminated. Another factor may be that, after a surgical approach to the heart, the clear pericardial fluid that normally inhabits the sac around the heart is no longer present, so that the heart in essence "sticks" to the surrounding tissues. This may produce a greater "torque" effect when the heart beats, the way that revving your car's engine will make the chassis of your vehicle roll several degrees.

Whatever the origin of this sensation, it will very likely not bother you in the long term. The sensation itself will dissipate. Also, you will become accustomed to the new feelings. No patient has ever voiced to us a persistent complaint about this sensation, which, once again, is not harmful in the slightest.

Can I get a stroke from my new artificial valve?

Despite treatment with Coumadin, some patients will develop blood clots on their valve that can *embolize*, or travel, to different parts of the circulatory tree. Most of these events are clinically silent; that is, we don't even know about them because the body compensates. However, when these small clots travel to the brain, they are usually clinically manifest. The patient may experience what we call a *TIA*, which stands for "transient ischemic attack." This medical terminology means a deprivation of blood flow that resolves spontaneously. This type of event is often called a mini-stroke. The symptoms can be any perturbation of function of the nervous system, usually involving disturbance of consciousness, speech, vision, sensation, or limb strength. If the symptoms resolve within twenty-four hours, we consider the event a mini-stroke, not a real stroke. If you ever feel any such symptoms, or if your family members detect any neurologic changes, your doctor should be contacted immediately.

Some patients may suffer a permanent stroke, in which symptoms similar to a TIA occur but fail to resolve within twenty-four hours. These can be very mild and barely detectable by the patient, or may be very severe, with a major impact on quality of life.

In general, there is about a 1 percent to 2 percent chance per year that a patient with an artificial aortic valve will develop a stroke or mini-stroke. For mitral valves, the rate is higher, at 3 percent to 4 percent. Again, keep in mind that many of these events are subtle or minor.

In general, keeping your INR (international normalized ratio; see chapter 9) in line will decrease your chance of having a valve-related complication. However, the INR is not the only factor. We know that the patient's general health plays a role. You should not smoke, since this will increase your chances of having an embolic event from your valve. Elderly patients with weak hearts and severe blood vessel disease are the most vulnerable to strokes from their heart valves. Young, otherwise healthy nonsmokers, are relatively safer.

What are the chances that my new heart valve will clot?

Very, very rarely, the artificial heart valve itself may clot, so that function of the leaflets is impaired. This is an emergency of the first order, as you may lapse quickly into profound heart failure or shock. Fortunately, such events are very rare. Valves in the aortic position are almost immune to this problem. Valves in the mitral position are almost exclusively vulnerable. For such an event to occur, there usually must be a major error in Coumadin assessment or dosage. This is the type of event that may occur if you do not take your Coumadin for days or weeks at a time. If such an event has indeed occurred, you will feel short of breath, weak, and light-headed. You should contact your doctor immediately or call an ambulance and go to the nearest emergency room. If you take your medications as prescribed, you should be overwhelmingly safe from the clotting of your valve.

Will I hear my valve?

You will not be able to hear an animal valve, as it is made of bio-logic tissue like your native valve and makes no audible noise when it closes. If you have a mechanical valve, you may be able to hear it if you are in a very quiet room and you have very good hearing. It is usually at night that the patient may hear the soft, stopwatch-like sound of a mechanical heart valve. We have *never* had a patient for whom this was a problem. Very likely you will become accustomed to this sound; in fact, most patients find it reassuring evidence that the heart and valve are working properly.

In earlier times, some mechanical valves produced quite loud closing sounds, which drew attention even when the patient, for example, entered a crowded elevator. These early-generation valves are no longer marketed in the United States (for reasons other than the noise effect).

I've been told that I will need antibiotics and will be at risk for infection after my valve is replaced. This bothers me. Can you explain this?

It is true that you must take antibiotics if you develop an infection after your new valve is placed. This could be a boil in your skin or an infection in your intestines or in your urinary or female tract. It is vitally important that you let your doctor know if you think you have such an infection so that you can be prescribed antibiotics to prevent "seeding" of your new valve by bacteria. As long as you responsibly report such events to your doctor and take the requisite antibiotics, you will in all probability be fine. Oral infections are special culprits. Be sure to let your dentist know that you have an artificial heart valve. In the case of coronary artery bypass patients, they have no foreign material in their bloodstream and therefore require no such antibiotic precautions.

Likewise, be sure to notify your surgeon if you are having invasive noncardiac surgery (or dental procedures) after your new heart valve is placed, so as to prevent any liberated bacteria from taking hold on your heart valve.

Lest these issues deter you from having a heart valve operation, remember that your native, diseased heart valve is similarly vulnerable to infection under similar circumstances to those described immediately above. Only normal, smooth, nondiseased valves are immune. In this respect, it is essentially a "wash" before and after operation—you are susceptible both with your own diseased valve and with your replacement valve. You should not allow these issues of valve infection to deter you from valve surgery if needed.

How will having a pacemaker change my life?

Having a pacemaker should have virtually no impact on your life or quality of life, except to make your life secure and relieve you of the constant concern that you could die from an abnormally low heart rate. The pacemaker should make you feel secure.

Of course, a pacemaker cannot prevent all causes of cardiac death. It can only prevent death from a heart rate that is too slow. Death can also result from a heart attack or from arrhythmia—a disturbed heart rhythm—usually an abnormally fast rhythm.

Also, a pacemaker will not improve the pumping strength of your heart. This is a common misconception.

Pacemakers are currently very small, often smaller than a silver dollar in diameter. The X-ray in the accompanying figure shows a pacemaker in place; note the fine wire running from the unit in the shoulder into the chamber of the heart. You will hardly be aware of the unit. The paced beats are not painful. You simply go on with your life.

You will be asked to report regularly, either in person or by phone, for checks on the condition of the battery in your pace-

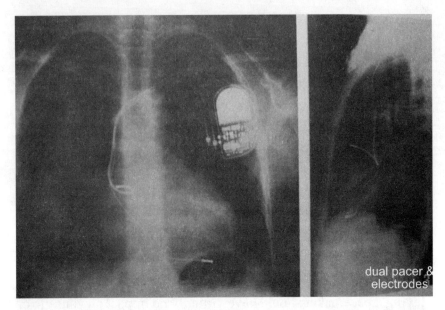

Figure 13.4. X-ray of transvenous pacemaker in place. Front and side views are shown.

maker. The battery life, although carefully monitored, is usually fine for ten years or more.

You do not have to worry about regular daily activities affecting your pacemaker. (Even being in close proximity to microwave ovens is generally not a problem, as long as the door closes properly.) Of course, if you work in the vicinity of heavy-duty equipment such as generators or power plants, these can affect the electrical function of your pacemaker. In such a circumstance, you would need to discuss the interaction of your environment and your pacemaker in detail with your doctor.

Chapter
14
HEART DISEASE IN WOMEN

Aren't women immune to heart disease?

Your question is a good one. To some extent, women are indeed protected against heart disease—especially the hardening of the arteries that so commonly affects men. This protection from hardening of the arteries of the heart—and, thus, from heart attack—extends from birth until menopause. It is extremely uncommon for a premenopausal woman to suffer from angina and/or a heart attack. In fact, women who fall prey to this disease early in life generally have juvenile onset diabetes or familial hyperlipidemia. With these diseases, the abnormalities of the arteries are so profound that even being a woman of childbearing age cannot confer sufficient protection.

However, after menopause, women catch up very quickly to men in terms of their likelihood of coronary artery disease. In fact, heart disease is the number one killer of postmenopausal women, outpacing even all cancers combined.[1] Moreover, while deaths from heart disease in men are decreasing, deaths from heart disease in women are actually *increasing*.[2] See figure 14.1. This is an epidemic that requires patient education, physician involvement, and dedicated cardiovascular research. African American women are especially prone to cardiovascular disease and heart-related death.

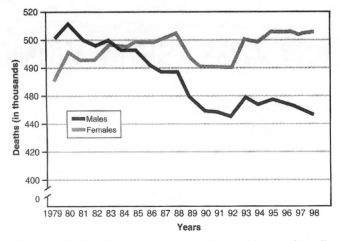

Figure 14.1. Graph showing the decrease in the incidence of cardiac death in men and the increase of cardiac death in women. Reprinted with permission from the American Heart Association.

Heart disease not only increases as women enter menopause, it is also more virulent in women than in men. Heart attacks lead more often to fatality in women than in men. Heart failure is more commonly fatal to women than to men.

While most women are aware of the dangers of breast and uterine cancer, fewer are cognizant of the critical toll exacted by coronary artery disease on women's lives.

So, you are correct that the female gender confers protection from heart disease, but only until about the early fifties, when menstruation typically ceases.

It is important to recognize that even being a woman does not protect against other forms of heart disease besides arteriosclerosis, such as congenital heart disease or valvular heart disease.

Please see the table 14.1 concerning heart disease in women.

Table 14.1. Myth versus Fact.

MYTH	FACT
Breast cancer is the leading cause of death in women.	While breast cancer claims forty-two thousand women each year, cardiovascular disease accounts for the deaths of five hundred thousand women annually. In fact, three times as many women die of heart disease each year as from all cancers combined. Virtually half of all female deaths are caused by heart disease.
Many more men die from heart disease than women.	More women die of heart attacks each year than men. This has been true since 1984.
Women tolerate surgery well.	The risk of death from cardiac surgery is significantly higher for women than for men. The same holds true for angioplasty and stenting.
All heart diseases are more common in men.	In fact, certain forms of heart disease predominate in women, including mitral valve prolapse, rheumatic fever, and ulcers of the aorta.
A heart attack is a heart attack.	A heart attack in a woman is more likely to be fatal than in a man.
A heart test is a heart test.	Actually, nuclear stress test results may be misleading for women, because the shadow of the left breast obscures visualization of the heart.

How does being a woman protect against arteriosclerosis?

Despite decades of concerted research, we still do not know the answer to this question. There is a general consensus that the hormones—estrogen—somehow prevent arteriosclerotic deposits in the arteries of the heart. We simply do not know how or why this is so. In fact, tremendous attention has been directed toward determining if giving estrogen treatment can extend the hormonal benefits into later stages of a woman's life. The simple answer is that this is not the case—hormone therapy after menopause is not protective against heart disease. In fact, for certain women, the risk of heart disease seems to be increased somewhat. A study conducted by the NIH (National Institute of Health) was actually terminated early because women on hormone therapy did more poorly than those without. Not only was the rate of heart attack higher, but the risks of stroke, blood clots, and breast cancer were elevated by hormone therapy (see figure 14.2).

One theory as to the mechanism by which women are protected has to do with the body's iron stores. Iron is essential for red blood cells, which carry oxygen to all parts of our body. However, it has been shown that iron contributes to the process of arteriosclerosis. Women generally have lower blood counts—fewer red blood cells and less iron in their bodies. This is because red blood cells and their contained iron are lost regularly each month with a woman's menstrual flow. Thus, it follows that men are at greater risk, and also that women lose their protection at menopause, when the monthly loss of iron ceases.

While in some ways an attractive concept, the iron hypothesis has never been proven conclusively.

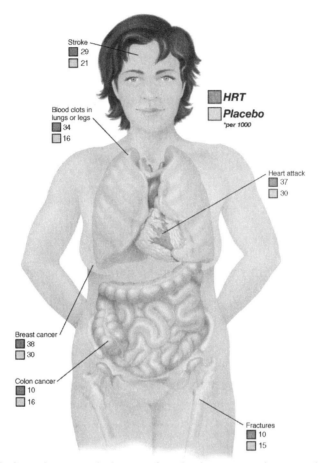

Figure 14.2. Organ by organ, the impact of routine hormone replacement therapy on a woman's health (from the NIH study). From *USA Today*, a division of Gannett Co., Inc. Reprinted with permission.

How about the "pill"? Is it really as bad as they say?

The vast majority of women can use a contraceptive pill without adverse consequences. There is no doubt, however, that the risk of cardiovascular problems is somewhat several times higher in women on the pill than in those not taking that form of contraception. Still, the likelihood of a problem occurring is on the order of one or two in ten thousand women on the pill.[3]

The problems that do occur tend to fall into two categories: First, women on the pill can manifest excess clotting in the veins, sometimes accompanied by passage of clots into the lungs (for pulmonary embolism, see the section titled "Why did the nurse ask me to flap my feet every hour?" in chapter 12). This usually occurs in the veins of the legs, where it is called *deep vein thrombosis* or DVT. Second, women on the pill can develop accelerated arteriosclerosis.

The risk of problems from the pill is higher in women over thirty-five years of age and women who smoke. Of course, diabetics and obese women are also at risk.

If you are a young, nonsmoking, trim, nondiabetic woman with no prior thrombosis or heart disease, it is perfectly reasonable for you to use the pill for contraception with your doctor's approval.

Does pregnancy affect a woman's heart?

Pregnancy most definitely has a major impact on the heart. The woman's circulatory system, by the end of pregnancy, is responsible for supplying blood and oxygen to a growing, newly developing human being in her womb. Also, the heart needs to supply the greater body mass of the woman as she gains weight. The amount of circulating blood nearly doubles by the end of the pregnancy, so the workload of the heart is doubled. The blood flow to the uterus increases from a trickle to more than a quart per minute. The blood flow to the breasts increases too. The blood flow to the skin increases by half again above normal, possibly as a means of dissipating heat. This situation is a strain on a normal heart, let alone a diseased heart. If a woman has underlying heart disease, usually of the valves, the heart may strain or fail during the course of pregnancy. Also, the high blood pressure that is common in the last trimester of pregnancy puts an additional burden on the heart. The circulatory changes that accompany pregnancy are depicted in figure 14.3.

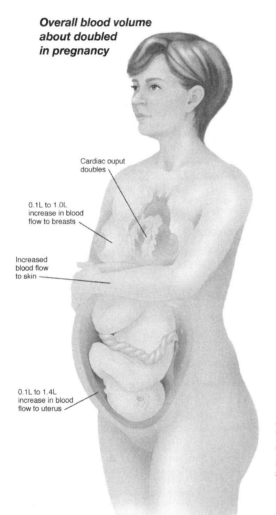

Overall blood volume about doubled in pregnancy

Cardiac ouput doubles

0.1L to 1.0L increase in blood flow to breasts

Increased blood flow to skin

0.1L to 1.4L increase in blood flow to uterus

Figure 14.3. The circulatory changes that accompany pregnancy.

If you know you have heart disease, you need to be monitored during your pregnancy not only by your gynecologist but also by a cardiologist. Sometimes you do not know you have heart disease until the extra burden of pregnancy unmasks cardiac symptoms.

The testing of your heart is somewhat limited in pregnancy, because of the fetus. We never wish to expose the fetus to the potential damaging influence of X-rays. Echocardiograms, however, are entirely safe. In fact, your baby will have many echo exams through your abdominal wall during the course of a normal pregnancy.

One very special and severe cardiac condition can occur during pregnancy—aortic dissection (see chapter 10). This tearing of the internal layers of the aorta is brought on by the added circulatory burden of advanced pregnancy, by the high blood pressure, and especially by the dramatic straining and bearing down needed for childbirth. Most women affected by this very serious condition—aortic dissection of pregnancy—are made vulnerable by an underlying aortic enlargement or weakening. If you have a history of aneurysms or dissections in your family, please bring this to the attention of your gynecologist. Special precautions need to be taken. Fortunately, peripartum aortic dissection is a rare phenomenon. We are called to see a case only once every year or two. When it does occur, it threatens both the mother and the baby.

How do the symptoms of heart attack differ in a woman compared to a man?

Our entire concept of angina and heart attack symptoms are based on what a male experiences. Recent attention has revealed that what a woman feels may be very different from what a man feels. Please see figure 14.4.

A woman may not feel the classic gripping pain in the central chest with radiation to the neck or left arm. She may feel only some vague sense of unease, perhaps accompanied by nausea, fatigue, jaw pain, weakness, or dizziness. Doctors often refer to such symptoms as *atypical* or deviating from the (male) norm. Not only may the woman herself not recognize the cardiac origin of her symptoms, but the diagnosis may also easily elude her physician. Heart disease presentation is much more subtle in women than in men.

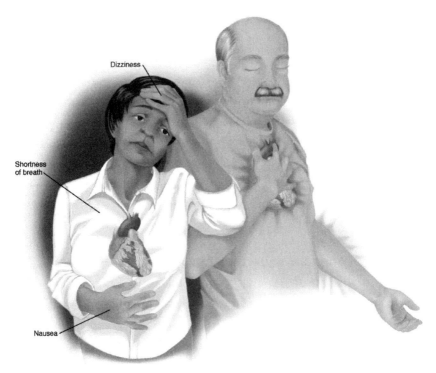

Dizziness

Shortness
of breath

Nausea

Figure 14.4. Comparison of how a heart attack may be perceived by women as opposed to men.

(Some might say that symptoms in women's hearts are more varied and complex, just like the adage that the neurological workings of a woman's brain are complicated and nuanced compared to those of a man.)

For this reason, especially if there is heart disease in the family, a woman with new symptoms, such as those described above, should be sure to seek evaluation. An EKG is certainly warranted. A stress test, often with echocardiographic enhancement or with nuclear images (see chapter 7) may be warranted. It is interesting to note that, even with nuclear imaging, the anatomy of a woman may make diagnosis more difficult, since the shadow of the left breast may obscure the heart.

Are any heart diseases more common in women?

Yes. Mitral valve prolapse (excess floppiness of the leaflets of the mitral valve) and rheumatic fever (an inflammation of the heart valves) are indeed significantly more common in women. You can learn more about these conditions in chapters 4 and 10, respectively.

I am still confused about the role of hormone replacement for women. Is it harmful or helpful?

The issue of hormone replacement therapy (HRT) is complex. For decades it was observed that premenopausal women had a lower incidence of heart disease than comparably aged men but that the incidence increased after menopause. It was believed that women were protected from developing heart disease by their estrogen. It seemed logical to assume that replacing estrogen in post-menopausal women would then confer a continuing resistance to their development of heart disease.

This hypothesis was tested in several clinical trials funded by the NIH. The first trial, the Heart and Estrogen/Progestin Replacement Study, or HERS, tested women who had previously suffered a heart attack.[4] Half of the group received estrogen replacement therapy and half received a placebo. This study found that the risk of a second heart attack was actually increased in the first year in those women taking hormone replacement.

The NIH started a large study in the late 1990s called the Women's Health Initiatives.[5] Over sixteen thousand post-menopausal women with no known prior heart disease were given either hormone replacement therapy or placebo. The trial was halted in 2002. The investigators found that the women who took hormones had an increased risk for breast cancer, stroke, and blood clots in the legs and lungs. Furthermore, they were not protected from heart disease overall. They were found to have fewer bone fractures and may have had a lower incidence of colorectal cancer. It should be noted, however, that the average age of the women in this study was sixty-four. This is about a decade above the average age when menopause begins.

In January 2006, the findings from the Nurses' Health Study, a large observational trial of women who started therapy soon after menopause, usually in their early fifties, reported a reduced risk of coronary artery disease—by a full 30 percent.[6] The benefit appeared to diminish the longer the women waited after menopause to initiate treatment.

These important trials suggest that hormone therapy is beneficial for the woman's heart when it is initiated early, during a narrow "window of opportunity" around the time of menopause, presumably before women build up atherosclerotic plaque. It is at just this time, at the beginning of menopause, that many women become symptomatic with hot flashes, drenching sweats, vaginal dryness, and insomnia. It is common for these symptoms to be totally alleviated by hormone replacement. The recent findings that hormone replacement may be beneficial for the heart, if started at an earlier stage of menopause, is particularly welcome news for this group of symptomatic women.

Thus, the bottom line is that there is no clear answer to the issue of hormone therapy, despite intensive investigations in large-scale, randomized clinical trials. Hormone replacement certainly improves the uncomfortable symptoms of menopause. If started early enough after onset of menopause, hormone replacement may confer some cardio-protective benefit. However, hormone therapy does increase the potential for development of clots in veins in susceptible women.

If you are a woman who wishes to take hormone therapy for treatment of menopausal symptoms, we would not disagree with your doing so. But you should, as with any medication, consult your own physicians before beginning such a regimen.

How do women tolerate cardiac surgery?

The bypass operation is generally easier to perform on a man than a woman. Women's tissues are flimsier, and the arteries—the microscopic target vessels to which the bypasses need to be sutured—are smaller, often much smaller.

These factors have led to a higher risk of death from the coronary bypass procedure in women than in men. The operation is still safe, but the risk is about 50 percent higher in women than in men. Recent studies have shown that it is actually body size that accounts for this risk. That is, women are smaller, have smaller arteries, and thus have higher surgical risk. Very small men also are at increased risk, and tall women are at less risk.

Also, for similar reasons, the long-term expectations—in terms of angina relief and survival—are somewhat blunted for women compared to men after coronary bypass surgery. Women's bypasses are not quite as durable as men's.

Surgery is still safe and effective—lifesaving in many instances—but not to the degree it is for men.

It is important to recognize that the same increased risk that women face with cardiac surgery also holds true for angioplasty and stenting of coronary heart disease in women[7] (see chapter 9). In fact, the risk of death after angioplasty is higher for women, as is the risk of closure of the artery after the angioplasty is performed.

How does a woman deal with the incision in the middle of her chest?

For extremely large-breasted women, the weight of the breasts themselves can pull against the incision. Wearing a brassiere, even immediately after surgery in the ICU, can help alleviate the skin tension and the accompanying discomfort.

Also, the *intertriginous folds*—the area under the breast where the breast tissue rubs against the skin of the chest—can be a source of problems. Moisture and excoriation in this region can lead to infection, even of the chest wound itself. It is important to maintain good hygiene in this area before the operation and to keep it clean and dry after surgery. Sometimes a small surgical dressing under each breast can help prevent rubbing of the skin.

Does harvesting the mammary artery for use in the bypass operation damage the breast?

The answer to this question is no. Although the mammary artery is named for the breast that it supplies with blood, no detriment ensues. The breast has an abundant network of blood vessels besides the mammary artery that continues to supply all the blood flow required by the breast even after the mammary artery has been "borrowed" for use on the heart (see chapter 12).

I don't want the incision down the middle of my chest. What other alternatives do I have?

This question comes up most often among young or unmarried women. This is understandable. These women may be having surgery for congenital heart disease or for valvular heart disease. The incision can show if a woman is wearing a bathing suit or shirt with an open collar. Many women are also concerned about what a boyfriend or husband may think.

For some women (usually young ones), because of these concerns, we use a submammary incision.[8] This incision hides in the creases under the breasts (see figure 14.5). It is hardly visible, even when the woman is naked. Even with such a horizontal incision, we can still open the breastbone vertically.

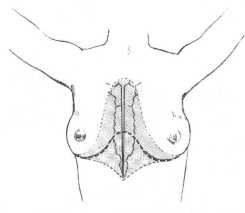

Figure 14.5. The submammary incision for major cardiac surgery in women. The scar hides in the crease under each breast, leading to improved appearance in and out of clothes. The traditional vertical incision is avoided.

While the submammary approach adds somewhat to the complexity of the operation, this is usually not a serious factor.

If you are concerned about a vertical scar, ask your surgeon about the submammary approach or other incisions that may be useful in your particular situation. Mitral valve surgery, for example, can be performed through a small incision confined to the region under your right breast.

Nothing is free in life however. The submammary approach can produce numbness in the nipple area. While this is often temporary, that is not always the case, and you should be aware of this possibility.

I heard on TV that my migraines are caused by a hole in my heart. How can this be?

You are correct that this possibility is being considered.

Migraines are extremely common in women. More than one in ten women are sufferers. It has very recently been noticed that patients with migraine headaches commonly have a small hole in the heart, which is called a *patent foramen ovale*. This is Latin for "small hole in the heart." It is a variant of *atrial septal defect*, which refers to a hole in the wall between the upper chambers of the heart, or atria (see figure 14.6).

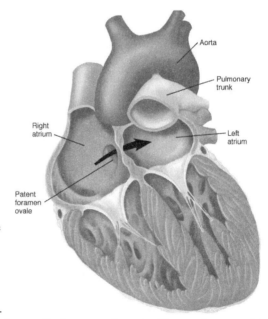

Figure 14.6. A *patent foramen ovale*—a small hole in the upper chambers of the heart—which may possibly be involved in causing migraines.

We do not understand exactly how such a small opening results in a migraine. It is presumed that small clots, originating in the legs after sitting or standing for a long time, pass through the small hole to reach the brain. In the brain, these small clots may cause spasms of the brain arteries, leading to the pain and other phenomena (auras and the like) characteristic of migraines.

In fact, so strong is the interest in patent foramen ovale as a cause of migraines, that a multicenter trial approved by the FDA has begun.[9] In affected women, the hole is closed by a small device passed through the veins, without an incision. This device is called an umbrella, because of its shape.

Within five or seven years, we should know if this form of treatment is truly effective for migraines, which burden and often incapacitate so many millions of women.

How will taking Coumadin affect my periods?

At times, young women who are still menstruating need to take Coumadin, usually because they need an artificial heart valve or because of thrombosis (clots), commonly in the leg veins.

You can expect your periods to be a bit heavier. But as long as your uterus is healthy, you should not have excessive bleeding from Coumadin.

If older women beyond menopause develop bleeding from the female tract while on Coumadin, this can indicate that there is an abnormality, even a tumor, in the uterus. The onset of bleeding from the female tract in a menopausal woman who is on Coumadin warrants a visit to the gynecologist.

Can I become pregnant on Coumadin?

Some young women of childbearing age require an artificial heart valve and need to be treated with Coumadin. For these women, becoming pregnant may be somewhat difficult, but it is definitely possible, and reasonably safe if done properly.

Nonetheless, Coumadin itself is not safe for a baby. Coumadin results in a high rate of miscarriage. Also, Coumadin is what we call *teratogenic*, or damaging to the fetus—highly so. It is simply not appropriate to take Coumadin during your pregnancy, especially the earlier phases.

So adjustments need to be made. Some women can go through pregnancy without Coumadin, often on aspirin alone. More commonly, we substitute the drug heparin for Coumadin. Heparin is not teratogenic. Also, heparin and heparinlike drugs do not cross the placenta, so the fetus is not directly exposed to these drugs. Heparin is safe for the baby's development in the uterus. The problem is that heparin cannot be taken orally but is given by subcutaneous injection, just like insulin is injected by diabetics. This is not too onerous once you are used to it. An alternate form of heparin, known as Lovenox, can be given at more widely spaced intervals, so you should not need to give yourself a shot more than once, or at most twice, a day.

This whole process is safer if your artificial valve is in the aortic position, where it is relatively safer from clots. If your valve is in the mitral position, the risk of forming clots on the valve is a bit higher. Still, with careful coordination between your obstetrician and your cardiologist, and a large measure of patience on your part, you can be carried through your pregnancy. The effort will be worthwhile when your new baby is placed on your lap after delivery.

Because of these issues related to Coumadin, many young women opt for biological valves instead of mechanical valves (see chapter 12). Biological valves do not require blood thinners, and so these Coumadin/pregnancy issues are obviated. However, the biological valve will wear out after about fifteen years, and another operation will be necessary.

AFTERWORD

I t is understandable that patients and their families might retain only some of the information given to them during visits with their doctors. There are many reasons for this. The material is often strange and highly technical. There is always high anxiety during important cardiac-related visits. The doctor may be in a hurry and may not always translate his medical jargon into a parlance understandable to patients and their families. The patient may be under the influence of anesthetic or sedative medications, especially if invasive procedures have been performed.

We hope that this book has provided you, in plain language and with the aid of illustrations and pictures, the background information on heart disease that you need. We hope that this information will be available as a resource that you can consult periodically, as necessary, without having to rely only on your memory. We hope that this book has answered many of your important questions and has also provided additional questions that you may wish to pose to your doctor.

Above all, we must emphasize the wisdom of the old adage that "a little knowledge can be a dangerous thing." This book is not intended to allow you to diagnose or treat yourself or to replace the crucial exchange of information between you and your physicians. The information in this book is intended only to supplement information provided in *your* visits with *your* doctors.

We hope that this book will aid you and your family in your pursuit of cardiac health. Our best wishes for a healthy future go out to all of our readers. Medical science stands ready to help you in achieving your optimal heart health.

GLOSSARY

Aneurysm A swelling of an artery, sometimes resembling the bulging of an old tube tire. *Aortic aneurysm* is a swelling, or enlargement, of the aorta—the main blood vessel of the body. Aneurysms are important because they can rupture.

Angina Pain in the chest caused by insufficient blood flow to the heart muscle. This pain is usually felt right behind the breastbone. It often produces a sensation of a crushing or pressurelike discomfort.

Angina at rest Chest pain that occurs without exertion or other provocation. This is a serious pattern of angina that requires prompt notification of your doctor.

Angioplasty The "plaque-busting" technique of inflating a balloon inside a coronary artery to relieve the narrowing. This is one of the techniques that can be done nonsurgically with a catheter in the catheterization laboratory.

Antiarrhythmic A drug used to combat an arrhythmia, or abnormal rhythm of the heart.

Aorta The large central artery that provides branches to supply blood to all organs of the body.

Aortic dissection A serious condition in which the wall of the aorta splits into two layers, creating a "double-barrel" aorta.

Aortic valve The main outflow valve of the heart. *Aortic stenosis* refers to narrowing of this valve. *Aortic regurgitation* refers to leaking of this valve.

Arrhythmia An abnormal rhythm of the heart.

Ascites The buildup of fluid in the abdomen, at times a manifestation of congestive heart failure. You may note an increase in your abdominal girth, or a swishing when you move around in bed.

Atrial septal defect A small hole in the membrane that divides the two upper chambers of the heart, or atria. This has recently been implicated in causing migraine headaches.

Atrium The upper chamber of each side of the heart. There is a right and a left atrium. These chambers serve to preload, or boost, the action of the vital lower chambers, or ventricles, of the heart.

Balloon pump A small mechanical device placed into the aorta to assist the heart function. The balloon passes through the femoral artery in the leg to reach its position just behind the heart. The balloon is a temporary device. This device takes a great burden off the heart and can relieve otherwise resistant angina pains. This device can also be used to support a heart that is struggling after open heart surgery.

Beta-blockers An important and powerful class of drugs that decrease the rate and forcefulness of the heartbeat. These drugs are especially useful in the treatment of angina and arrhythmias.

Bradycardia A slow heart rate, defined as one below sixty beats per minute. This can cause dizziness or loss of consciousness.

Calcium channel blockers An important and powerful class of drugs that dilate the arteries of the heart, helping to get more blood to the heart muscle. They also dilate the arteries of the body, lowering blood pressure and relieving the workload of the heart. These drugs can furthermore decrease the heart rate, helping to treat arrhythmias.

Cardiomyopathy Weakening of the heart muscle. The term comes from the Greek "cardia," or *heart*, and "pathia," or *weakness*. Cardiomyopathy is called *ischemic* if it results from heart attacks or *idiopathic* if it is of unknown cause.

Catheterization An essential type of cardiac test in which wires and tiny tubes are passed into the heart to permit measurement of pressures in the heart, visualization of the strength and contraction pattern of the heart, and detailed assessment of the coronary arteries for possible blockages. This is the "gold standard" of cardiac diagnostic tests.

Collateral circulation Enlarged secondary tributaries that arise in response to blockage of main arteries. These tributaries run parallel to the blocked arteries, providing some measure of blood flow to the starved heart muscle beyond the blockage points.

Congestive heart failure A state of excess fluid in the lungs and legs, due to backup of water behind weak pumping chambers of the heart. There are many possible causes of this problem.

Coronary artery One of the small arteries that run on the surface of the heart and provide nourishment to the heart muscle. It is the coronary arteries that become blocked and cause heart attacks.

Coumadin A powerful blood thinning medication. Another name for this drug is Warfarin. It is used for patients with mechanical heart valves or with atrial fibrillation.

Defibrillator The paddle device used to convert dangerous heart rhythms to normal ones by powerful electrical discharge.

Diastole The passive filling phase of the cardiac cycle, in which the powerful ventricles wait passively, preparing for the active contraction to come.

Dyspnea Medical term for "shortness of breath."

Echocardiogram or "echo" A test using sound waves, like sonar, to obtain images of your heart. This test can disclose problems with the valves of your heart or with the pumping strength of your heart. It is a comfortable and easy test to take. At times, your doctor may order or perform a transesophageal echocardiogram, in which the echo probe is passed through your throat into the esophagus, or swallowing tube. This type of echo gives superb images of your heart, as the probe lies just behind the heart inside your body.

Edema The medical term for swelling from water retention. This is usually manifested in the ankles. It can be a sign of heart failure, as well as other physical problems. The edema may show an imprint if you press your thumb against the swollen skin.

Ejection fraction A measure of the pumping strength of the left ventricle, the most important pumping chamber of the heart. This value represents the proportion of blood ejected with each heartbeat. A normal value is 70 percent. If ejection fraction falls below 40 percent, then symptoms of inadequate pumping strength of the heart may appear.

Electrocardiogram or EKG An electrocardiogram, or test of the electrical signals of your heart. This is a simple and easy test, which can show evidence of inadequate blood flow to the heart, heart attack, or abnormal rhythm of the heart.

Electrophysiologic (or EP) test A test for patients with a history of or who may be at risk for severe cardiac arrhythmia. The test is done by tickling the heart electrically via a catheter passed into the chambers of the heart.

Embolus (also embolism) A traveling particle in the bloodstream. This is often a particle of arteriosclerotic debris or clot. In the systemic circulation, this may be devastating if the particle travels to the heart (coronary arteries) or to the brain. On the pulmonary side of the circulation, these particles may go to the lung (pulmonary embolism), causing difficulty breathing or even shock and death.

Endocarditis Infection of a heart valve, which is a type of bloodstream infection. This is a serious problem that can destroy the valve tissue. Antibiotics and/or surgery are always required.

Endocardium The innermost of the three layers of the heart wall. This layer is the most susceptible and first to be affected in a heart attack.

Epicardium The outermost layer of the heart wall. This is the last to be affected by a heart attack.

Fibrillation A fast, chaotic heart rhythm. Ventricular fibrillation, affecting the powerful lower heart chambers, is a very serious rhythm disturbance that invariably causes cardiac arrest. Atrial fibrillation, affecting the upper chambers of the heart, is more common and much more benign.

Functional A term describing an innocent murmur, one occurring in a normally functioning valve. This can also be described as an "innocent" murmur.

Heart-lung machine The mechanical device that takes over the functions of the heart and the lungs while the most intricate segments of open heart surgery are performed. It includes a pump to circulate the blood and an artificial lung. The heart-lung machine is colloquially called, in professional circles, simply, "the pump."

Heart murmur An abnormal sound heard through a stethoscope, representing turbulent flow across a dysfunctional heart valve. A murmur may be present because of either narrowing or leaking of the affected valve.

Heparin A powerful blood thinner, usually given intravenously, especially for blood clots, heart attacks, or artificial heart valves. This drug is especially useful because it wears off within two to four hours, unlike oral blood thinners, which can take days to dissipate.

Holter monitor A continuous tape recording of your EKG done by a portable machine while you go about your daily life. This is used to look for arrhythmias—abnormal heart rhythms—which may not be detected on a "spot" EKG while you are in the doctor's office.

Hypertension High blood pressure. This is defined as a pressure exceeding 140/90 millimeters of mercury.

Hypertrophy A state in which the main pumping chamber of the heart—the left ventricle—becomes thick and muscle-bound from pressure overload. This is a harmful condition.

Inflammation The medical term for irritation of tissues. This irritation may be from infection or from noninfectious causes. Many authorities feel that inflammation is an important cause of arteriosclerosis and coronary artery disease.

Internal mammary artery The artery that runs inside the chest wall just beside the breastbone. It gets its name because it normally supplies blood to the breast. We "borrow" this artery for use in supplying blood to the heart. This artery is the most durable conduit for the coronary artery bypass operation.

Mitral valve The main inflow valve of the heart. Mitral stenosis refers to narrowing of this valve. Mitral regurgitation refers to leaking of this valve.

Myocardial infarction The technical term for a heart attack, or death of a portion of the heart muscle. This is usually caused by blockage of one of the coronary arteries, which supply blood and oxygen to the heart muscle.

Myocardium The thick, middle layer of the heart wall. This contains the millions of heart muscle cells that actually do the job of producing a mechanical heartbeat.

Myxoma A fairly common type of tumor arising in the heart. It usually occurs in the left atrium. Surgery is required and is often curative.

Pericardial constriction A disease state in which the heart sac becomes thick, rigid, and tight. It squeezes the heart so that effective pumping strength is impaired.

Pericardial effusion The fluid that resides in the pericardial space that lubricates the heart's functions. A small amount of fluid is normally present. Larger amounts, found in disease states, can compromise heart function.

Pericardial tamponade A disease state in which the heart sac is filled with an abnormally large amount of fluid (or blood), compromising heart function significantly. In essence, the fluid squeezes the heart so badly that the heart cannot pump effectively. Circulatory problems up to and including shock and death can occur.

Pericardiectomy Surgical removal of the pericardial sac, necessary in cases of severe pericardial disease.

Pericardiocentesis Drawing off of pericardial fluid by needle.

Pericardium The thin, glistening, flexible but inelastic (nonstretchable) sac that surrounds the heart in its central position in the chest.

Prolapse Excess backward movement of a heart valve leaflet. Usually applied to the mitral valve. Mitral valve prolapse can often be a completely benign, or mild, condition.

Pulmonary edema A state of flooding of the lungs with fluid backed up behind a weak heart. Shortness of breath is usually profound. This is a very serious manifestation of congestive heart failure.

Regurgitation Backward leakage through a heart valve.

Rheumatic fever An infection, usually occurring during childhood or early adulthood, which can affect the heart and heart valves. Problems with valve function may occur years later, in adult life. Rheumatic fever may follow untreated sore throats, caused by the streptococcus bacterium.

Stenosis A narrowing, as in an artery or a cardiac valve.

Stent The fine metal "fencing" often used to supplement an angioplasty procedure. The stent stays permanently inside the stretched artery, serving to keep the blockage from pushing its way again into the open channel of the artery.

Stress test A test in which a stress is placed on your heart, either by having you exercise or by giving you a powerful medication. This test is used to screen for blocked coronary arteries or to assess the impact of known blockages. During this test, the doctor will check to see if you are feeling chest pain, if your EKG changes, or if images taken by nuclear or echo means show any abnormalities. The exercise for this test is usually performed on a treadmill, thus many doctors refer to this as the "treadmill test."

Syncope The medical term for fainting.

Systole The active phase of cardiac contraction, during which the powerful ventricles eject blood from the heart.

Thrill A vibration felt by the examiner's hand placed over the heart in cases with very loud heart murmurs. The presence of a thrill represents intensely turbulent flow across a very abnormal heart valve.

Thrombolytic A type of drug used to treat an evolving heart attack. These drugs are the "clot busters," which actually dissolve existing clots in the coronary artery.

Transmural myocardial infarction A heart attack that goes all the way through the heart wall. This is more extensive and more serious than a nontransmural heart attack.

Unstable angina Angina of increasing pattern, occurring more frequently, lasting longer, requiring more nitro pills for control, or even occurring without exertion or other provocation. Unstable angina may presage a heart attack and should be promptly reported.

Vegetation A collection, or clump, of infected material, including bacteria and debris, on the surface of a heart valve. This can be seen in valve infections referred to as "endocarditis."

Ventricle The lower pumping chamber of each side of the heart. There is a right and a left ventricle. These are the important pumping chambers of the heart.

LIST OF CASE VIGNETTES

5.1	Grandma Maria	Hypertension and stroke	"Maria from Italy"
5.2	Arnold Kramer	Hypertension and kidney failure	"High Blood Pressure and Low Kidney Function"
5.3	Thirty-seven-year old runner	Juvenile diabetes and premature coronary disease	"The Devastation of Juvenile Diabetes"
5.4	Mr. Amarante	Diffuse arteriosclerosis	"Arteriosclerosis Everywhere"
9.1	Mr. Fulton	Mechanical heart	"Playing the Odds"
10.1	Angela, the author's date	Rheumatic fever— contagious?	"Your Author's Girlfriend"
10.2	Carmella, the professor's wife	Aortic dissection	"The Professor's Wife"
10.3	Selma from Brazil	Cardiac tumor	"The Girl from Ipanema"
12.1	The cardiologist	Constrictive pericarditis	"A Colleague in Trouble"

LIST OF ILLUSTRATIONS AND TABLES

INTRODUCTION

CHAPTER 1

CHAPTER 2

CHAPTER 3

CHAPTER 8

CHAPTER 9

CHAPTER 10

CHAPTER 11

CHAPTER 12

CHAPTER 13

NOTES

CHAPTER 3: ARRHYTHMIAS

1. J. L. Cox, "Surgical Treatment of Atrial Fibrillation: A Review," supplement 1, nos. 20–9. *Europace* (2004): 5.

2. R. Fountain and others, "The PROTECT AF (WATCHMAN Left Atrial Appendage System for Embolic PROTECTion in Patients with Atrial Fibrillation) Trial," *American Heart Journal* 5 (2006): 956–61.

CHAPTER 5: HYPERTENSION, HIGH CHOLESTEROL, AND ARTERIOSCLEROSIS

1. Adapted with permission from P. Libby and P. M. Ridker, "Inflammation and Atherosclerosis: Role of C-reactive Protein in Risk Assessment," *American Journal of Medicine* 116 (2004): 9S–16S.

2. P. W. Ewald, *Plague Time: The New Germ Theory of Disease* (Free Press, 2002).

3. F. Yusuf, Reported in Interheart study. This discussion is adapted from an excellent article in *USA TODAY*, January 9, 2006. The primary scientific report appeared in *Lancet* (September 11–17, 2004): 937–52.

CHAPTER 8: LIVING WITH HEART DISEASE: LIFESTYLE CHANGES THAT PROTECT YOUR HEART

1. G. A. Bray and D. S. Gray, "Obesity. Part I—Pathogenesis," *Western Journal of Medicine* 149 (1988): 429–41.

2. Body mass index chart from http://www.consumer.gov/weight-loss/bmi.htm, adapted with permission from Bray and Gray, "Obesity."

CHAPTER 9: TREATMENT: MEDICATIONS, THERAPIES, AND PROCEDURES

1. C. Gardiner and others, "Patient Self-Testing Is a Reliable and Acceptable Alternative to Laboratory INR Monitoring," *British Journal of Haematology* 128 (2005): 242–47.

2. P. Y. Liu and others, "Androgens and Cardiovascular Disease," *Endocrine Reviews* 24 (2003): 313–40; "An Evaluation of Estrogenic Substances in the Treatment of Cerebral Vascular Disease," Report of the Veterans Administration Cooperative Study of Atherosclerosis, Neurology Section, *Circulation* 33 (1966): 3–9.

3. A. Keech and others, "Effects of Long-Term Fenofibrate Therapy on Cardiovascular Events in 9795 People with Type 2 Diabetes Mellitus (The FIELD Study): Randomized Controlled Trial," *Lancet* 26, no. 366 (2005): 1849–61.

4. FDA Talk Paper, T01-34. August 8, 2001. Print Media: 301-827-6242. Consumer Inquiries: 888-INFO-FDA, http://www.fda.gov/bbs/topics /ANSWERS/2001/ANS01095.html.

5. J. M. Gaziano and C. M. Gibson, "Potential for Drug-Drug Interactions in Patients Taking Analgesics for Mild-to-Moderate Pain and Low-Dose Aspirin for Cardioprotection," *American Journal of Cardiology* 97, no. 9A (2006): 23–29.

6. S. Prakash and V. Valentine, "Timeline: The Rise and Fall of Vioxx," NPR archives, http://www.npr.org/templates/story/story.ho?storyId=5470430.

7. P. K. Kuchalakanti and others, "Correlates and Long-Term Outcomes of Angiographically Proven Stent Thrombosis with Sirolimus- and Paclitaxel-eluting Stents," Circulation 113 (2006): 1108–13; J. A. Spertus and others, "Prevalence, Predictors, and Outcomes of Premature Discontinuation of Thienopyridine Therapy After Drug-Eluting Stent Place-

ment," Results from the PREMIER Registry, Circulation, http://circ.aha-journals.org/cgi/content/full/113/24/2803.

8. Adapted with permission from J. A. Franciosa and others, "Survival in Men with Severe Chronic Left Ventricular Failure Due to Either Coronary Heart Disease or Idiopathic Dilated Cardiomyopathy." *American Journal of Cardiology* 51 (1983): 831–36.

9. R. Sunderji and others, "Pulmonary Effects of Low Dose Amiodarone; A Review of the Risks and Recommendations for Surveillance," *Canadian Journal of Cardiology* 16 (2000): 1435–40; L. A. Siddoway, "Amiodarone: Guidelines for Use and Monitoring," *American Family Physician* 11 (2003): 2189–96.

CHAPTER 12: SURGICAL PROCEDURES

1. B. W. Lytle, "Prolonging Patency: Choosing Coronary Bypass Grafts," *New England Journal of Medicine* 351 (2004): 2262–54.

2. D. Kumar and others, "Anticoagulation in Patients with Prosthetic Heart Valves," *Cardiac Surgery Today* 2, no. 1 (2004): 126–33.

3. J. A. Elefteriades and I. L. Kron, "CABG in Advanced Left Ventricular Dysfunction," *Cardiology Clinics* 13 (1995): 35–42.

4. J. Cai and P. I. Terasaki, "Heart Transplantation in the United States 2004," *Clinical Transplants* (2004): 31–34.

CHAPTER 14: HEART DISEASE IN WOMEN

1. L. Mosca and others, "Cardiovascular Disease in Women: A Statement for Healthcare Professionals from the American Heart Association," *Circulation* 96 (1997): 2468–82.

2. American Heart Association, 2001 Heart/Stroke Statistical Update.

3. L. A. Gillum and others, "Ischemic Stroke Risk with Oral Contraceptives: A Meta-analysis," *Journal of the American Medical Association* 284 (2000): 72–78.

4. S. Hulley and others, "Randomized Trial of Estrogen Plus Progestin for Secondary Prevention of Coronary Heart Disease in Postmenopausal Women," Heart and Estrogen/Progestin Replacement Study (HERS) Research Group, *Journal of the American Medical Association* 19 (1998): 605–13.

5. G. L. Anderson and others, "Effects of Conjugated Equine Estrogen in Postmenopausal Women with Hysterectomy: The Women's Health Initiative Randomized Controlled Trial," *Journal of the American Medical Association* 291 (2004): 1701–12.

6. Personal communication (LSC).

7. W. S. Weintraub and others, "Percutaneous Transluminal Coronary Angioplasty in Women Compared to Men," *Journal of the American College of Cardiology* 24 (1994): 81–90; Paolo Angelini, "Percutaneous Transluminal Coronary Angioplasty," in *Heart Disease in Women*, ed. S. Wilansky and J. T. Willerson (New York: Churchill Livingston, 2002).

8. H. Laks and G. L. Hammond, "A Cosmetically Acceptable Incision for the Median Sternotomy," *Journal of Thoracic Cardiovascular Surgery* 79 (1980): 46–49.

9. B. Azarbal and others, "Association of Interatrial Shunts and Migraine Headaches: Impact of Transcatheter Closure," *Journal of the American College of Cardiology* 45 (2005): 489–92.

INDEX